Compassion and Caring in Nursing

Compassion and Caring in Nursing

CLAIRE CHAMBERS
*Leader, Specialist Community Public Health Nursing and
Community Specialist Practice Programmes
Oxford Brookes University*

and

ELAINE RYDER
*Formerly, Leader of the Community Specialist Practice Nursing Programme
Oxford Brookes University*

Foreword by

SARAH H KAGAN PhD, RN
*Professor of Gerontological Nursing
University of Pennsylvania, USA*

Radcliffe Publishing
Oxford • New York

Radcliffe Publishing Ltd
18 Marcham Road
Abingdon
Oxon OX14 1AA
United Kingdom

<u>www.radcliffe-oxford.com</u>
Electronic catalogue and worldwide online ordering facility.

British Library Cataloguing in Publication Data

A catalogue record for this book is available from the British Library.

ISBN-13: 978 184619 287 6

The paper used for the text pages of this book
is FSC certified. FSC (The Forest Stewardship
Council) is an international network to promote
responsible management of the world's forests.

FSC

Mixed Sources
Product group from well-managed
forests and other controlled sources
www.fsc.org Cert no. SGS-COC-2482
© 1996 Forest Stewardship Council

Typeset by Pindar NZ, Auckland, New Zealand
Printed and bound by TJI Digital, Padstow, Cornwall, UK

Contents

Foreword

I panicked for a long moment . . . Compassion? And caring? In nursing? What is there that can be new to say about compassion and caring? Too many doubts ran through my head a few hours after I had replied to Claire Chambers and Elaine Ryder that I would write a foreword for their upcoming book. I must be honest and admit that I first agreed to write this foreword on the strength of my collegial connection to Claire and Elaine. Then I had second thoughts about the topic. The risks were manifold; this is a topic too easily made trite or saccharine without conveying any real knowledge. To admit my reaction to the looming task of the foreword of this book to its readers – drawn by the title, the authors, or both – feels almost heretical. After all, admitting trepidation about exploring a topic so often associated with nurses and the discipline of nursing the world over is not something to confess lightly. My concerns have accrued over time. Compassion and caring, like advocacy and cultural sensitivity, are increasingly used with few substantive anchors in discussions of nursing. They have become the 'buzzwords' of our discipline, flying past our ears scarcely heard and their precise meanings lost.

Many American students and nurses who are young in practice describe themselves as the *advocate* who *cares* for the **patient**. Imbedded in that statement are the isolationist assumptions that nurses alone advocate and care for people. Personhood is simultaneously stripped away from those people with the exclusive label 'patient'. Care and – by implication – compassion provided by colleagues of other disciplines is rendered null and void. In advancing these assumptions, substantive content and analytic frames to support compassion and caring in advocacy, sensitivity and other myriad actions are most often neglected or even intentionally omitted. Compassion and caring become values that need no justification or analysis in order to be included in nursing. We claim them for ourselves alone.

People in need of nursing deserve and require compassion and care from those nurses. If people – individuals, families, even communities – are the object and subjects of nursing, then claims to compassion and care are for them and not for nursing. My dear colleague, Sandra Borton, who began her practice about the time I was born, is fond of saying that nursing is the only discipline in which identity is a verb. 'Nurses nurse', Sandy would say, and she has legions of protégés who quote that maxim to the nurses they now teach, instruct and mentor. Sandy's maxim is too often overshadowed by concerns that there is too much else to know to be a nurse today. Discourse about what it is exactly to be a nurse and how one embodies that state of being rarely surfaces against arguments about what new science must be added to basic curricula and continuing education. I respond to these arguments with the notion that nurses in practice today and those we educate for tomorrow do indeed need justification and analysis of the compassion and care they are to embody for the people whom they nurse. Science alone, applied from our own research and from that of other relevant disciplines, is insufficient. Nursing requires a larger, universal and lasting frame.

Nursing appears incredibly contextual in today's world. Where you nurse determines who is a nurse and what you perceive to be nursing. Knowledge of biomedicine and facility in coordinating highly technical medical care are much valued in developed and post-industrial societies. Using foundational knowledge of health, disease, injury and behaviour, while employing any available resources, combine to create an image of nursing in communities or societies where healthcare systems are inequitable and disparities persist. Yet, I have found, in meetings with colleagues – like Claire and Elaine – around the world, a universal connection among nurses; a connection that transcends national policies, role interpretation, and scope of practice. Does connection lie in a shared language rooted in understanding that nurses do indeed nurse? We must explore precisely how nurses nurse if this connection is true at all. Absent substantive exploration, and threats to any possible universality will quickly emerge. Nursing risks being too weak to withstand demands of a world where healthcare is an increasingly scarce and precious commodity, and the shortfall of available nurses escalates.

The compassion nurses have for those whom they nurse, and the care delivered in the context shaped by compassion, mandate analysis. How do nurses conceive of compassion? How and why do nurses integrate caring into practice? Where are compassion and caring situated in the relationship a nurse has with the person or people who receive that care? These are puzzling, intricate questions with often difficult but potentially powerful, evocative answers. Successful answers evoke frames and structures that anchor nursing in the present, offering paths to create nursing practice specific to the individual, family, and community in context. Claire Chambers and Elaine Ryder anchor nursing in a deceptively accessible and clearly practical analysis of compassion and caring *in* nursing. From the first chapter, they turned my trepidation into hope for nurses and nursing. My moment of panic became engagement and then satisfaction with chapter after carefully constructed chapter.

In a compelling reflection on the best in nursing, *Compassion and Caring in Nursing* is a pellucid synthesis of evidence and analysis of the elements of compassion and the creation of caring in nursing. Lucidity here stems largely from case studies that are at once very real and yet easily deciphered. Their well-chosen, scholarly sources for discussion create a sense of a global nursing epistemology, avoiding narrow regional or national understandings of compassion and caring. Claire and Elaine achieve remarkable clinical accessibility while maintaining rigorous scholarly evaluation as they combine case studies with evaluation to pose critical questions to the reader. This is a book every nurse and student nurse will want on the shelf closest at hand, to be opened at those moments of reflection where challenges to find compassion and questions of caring might overwhelm if not for the engagement of colleagues like Claire and Elaine.

Sarah H Kagan PhD, RN
Ralston House Term Professor of Gerontological Nursing,
School of Nursing
Clinical Nurse Specialist, Abramson Cancer Center
Secondary Faculty, Department of Otorhinolaryngology:
Head and Neck Surgery
University of Pennsylvania
Philadelphia, PA
January 2009

I am greatly thankful to Cheryl Boberick RN, Sandra Borton RN, Mary Denno MSN, RN, and Nancy Rodenhausen MA, RN for our long-standing dialogue about nurses and nursing. I am deeply grateful for conversation with Alicia A Puppione MSN, RN and Christine Ray MSW, in preparing this foreword.

Preface

We wanted to write this book because we have had a great deal of experience of students revisiting core concepts of nursing for their roles within community practice. This has been challenging and has significantly improved the practice of not only newly qualified nurses, but also those who are highly experienced in their field. We have seen an increase in anecdotal accounts that reflect a decrease in fundamental aspects of care, and we have felt strongly that nursing is in danger of losing its essence of caring. People are very clear about what they feel they need from current nursing practice and we wanted to work from the perspective of what patients, clients and carers actually value. We feel that compassion, in its many manifestations, is the key to rediscovering what lies at the heart of nursing practice all over the world. We feel it is absolutely essential that nurses start to revisit compassion as a central focus for nursing practice, and hope that this book will challenge nurses to think about their practice from the perspective of the patient. We hope that this book will be helpful to nurses, wherever they practise in the world, and whether they practise in primary, secondary or tertiary settings. Through this, we hope to improve the experience of patients and their friends and relatives.

We have planned this book to be as accessible and user friendly as possible. The focus is on the integration of theory and practice throughout. We want readers to be challenged by the points for reflection in terms of their own practice, and recognise the dilemmas raised within the case studies. We hope that this style of writing will encourage practitioners to review their current practice and bring about change within their working environment.

For us, compassion is the key to nursing and we wanted to be clear about what this means, and the challenges it brings in current nursing practice. We have focused on what we believe is central to compassionate care, namely:

- empathy and sensitivity
- dignity and respect
- listening and responding
- diversity and cultural competence
- choice and priorities
- empowerment and advocacy.

Each chapter focuses on two related aspects of compassionate practice and we have used case studies to generate discussion and create points to challenge practitioners in their nursing care.

Claire Chambers
Elaine Ryder
January 2009

About the authors

Claire Chambers MSc, PgDip (Prof) Ed, CPT, HV (Dip), RGN
Claire has worked as a nurse within various hospital environments in the UK and then moved into health visiting. She was a health visitor, community practice teacher and lecturer practitioner before she moved into full-time education. During her teaching career she worked with pre-registration students and then with postqualification and postgraduate students from various community and acute settings, but her prime interests have always been in relation to community practice. Patient- and client-centred care, diversity and cultural competence, public health and caring for people with long-term conditions are her special interests, with a particular emphasis on the importance of communication skills.

Elaine Ryder MSc, BA, DNT, RNT, Cert Ed, CPT, DN, RGN
Elaine has had appointments within different parts of the UK, as a district nurse, community practice teacher, manager and educator within primary care. Her particular experience and interest is in meeting the needs of vulnerable people and their carers at home; for example older people, people with long-term conditions, palliative care, or end-of-life needs as well as caring for those with acute healthcare needs at home.

Acknowledgements

We would like to thank those who have inspired us to write this book, our patients, clients and carers. Our students have always motivated us and stimulated debate. Their sensitive understanding of issues in different areas of practice has helped us think more deeply about compassion and what this means for practice. Our colleagues, throughout our careers in nursing, health visiting and teaching, have also been integral to our value system.

We would like to thank Gillian Nineham and the team at Radcliffe Publishing Ltd for their support and encouragement throughout the writing of this book. Also, we are very grateful to Professor Sarah Kagan for her spontaneous positive response to our request to write the foreword to this book. We would particularly like to thank Linda Fildew and Liz Cornish for their specific expertise. We have also found the patient opinion forum on www.patientopinion.org.uk highly helpful in accessing real life patient opinions and perspectives.

From a personal point of view, we would like to thank all those who have been so encouraging about our writing. We would like to thank our parents who have made us the people we are: Jack and Nancy Ephgrave and Ken and Monica Hale. In particular, we would like to thank the following people for their ongoing interest, encouragement and love: Irene, Amanda, Adrienne and Robert as well as Dannii, Jessica, Chris, Jonathan, Amy and Anna.

Our special thanks to Alan Chambers and Malcolm Ryder, our ever-supportive husbands, who have been so encouraging and constructive in the help they have given in their different ways. They have been very much a part of this process, and are very proud of our achievements. Their unfailing support has helped us maintain our motivation throughout the writing of this book.

CHAPTER 1

Introduction: Compassion in nursing – the key to caring

Overview of the chapter

Key theme one – compassion

- Case study
- Discussion
- What does compassion mean to patients and clients?
- Case study
- Discussion
- Thoughts for your practice
- How do nurses perceive compassion in their practice?
- Case study
- Discussion
- Thoughts for your practice

Key theme two – caring

- Case study
- Discussion
- Do we understand the importance of caring in nursing practice?
- Case study
- Discussion
- Thoughts for your practice
- How do we build caring relationships with individuals?
- Case study
- Discussion
- Thoughts for your practice
- Summary – links to compassion and caring
- References

OVERVIEW OF THE CHAPTER

Compassion is the essence of caring, and therefore the essence of nursing, in our opinion, and yet it is not always the central focus of nursing practice. This book has been written in an attempt to reintroduce the concept of compassion and caring into how we, as nurses, think about our practice and our patients and clients. We not only need to challenge ourselves to show more compassion towards those in our care, but also we need to challenge our colleagues and stimulate discussion with our students to ensure that compassion remains central in our nursing care.

There are many different definitions of compassion, but we strongly believe that it is demonstrated most clearly by acting in a way that you would like others to act towards you. We need to reach out to others with kindness through what we say and by our physical actions. We believe that compassion is a profound feeling, which is brought about by witnessing the pain or distress of others. However, nurses can feel vulnerable by witnessing others' distress and, therefore, may want to minimise this vulnerability by distancing themselves from the patient or client in distress. After all, if we can believe that the patient's experience is unique and could never happen to us, then we feel less at risk and more in control of our lives. This distancing of ourselves compromises our ability to be compassionate.

Wilkinson (2007) discusses the acculturation that nursing practice areas can adopt where there is an institutionalised heartlessness. This heartlessness is exemplified by ignoring the needs of patients and reinforcing to others, who work in that environment, that this is acceptable nursing practice. There is a lack of conscience and kindness, and a sense of duty to others is missing. As nurses, we need to ensure that there is a positive culture within our practice areas where tenderness and empathy are paramount. It is only then that we can truly demonstrate our compassion.

There is a growing amount of anecdotal evidence that nursing standards, in relation to compassion, are slipping. Procedures and interventions are being perceived by patients to be taking priority over patient care. Nurses are rushed, unsmiling and perfunctory, not caring or empathetic. Nurses are not being perceived necessarily as patient-focused. There have been criticisms of nurses discussing their social lives while patients are present, rather than engaging in communication with the patient. Examples from patient forums and other written sources will be used throughout the book to demonstrate good nursing practice, and where nursing is perceived to be falling short as a compassionate and caring profession.

Gadsby (2008) tells of her experience as a nurse unexpectedly thrust into the position of being a relative of someone who suddenly becomes acutely unwell. She says that, in retrospect, she was impressed with how well-trained the nurses actually were who cared for her relative, and how good they were at their jobs. However, she also says how hard it was to be on the other side of the fence, and how powerless she felt. She said that there did not appear to be the time or inclination on the part of the nurses to get to know her relative or the family, or to answer their questions. She says:

> How many of us, working with patients day after day, get used to not seeing the person behind the patient? How easy do we find it to focus on the task we have to do next, rather than pausing for a moment to check that the person we are with is not desperate to share anxieties or ask questions? I felt vulnerable and unsure, and I am used to the workings of a hospital ward. How much harder must it be for those who do not work in and understand the system? In the midst of being busy, let's all try to be still for long enough for those in our care and their loved ones to catch up with us and help us to see who they are, and to share something of ourselves with them. (Gadsby 2008, p. 8)

This is a valuable point. If we are constantly concentrating on the next task rather than who the patient is, we cannot be compassionate carers. Therefore, this introductory chapter will focus on compassion and caring as distinct entities in their own right, as well as how they become integral to the whole concept of compassionate care in nursing.

KEY THEME ONE – COMPASSION

CASE STUDY 1.1

Joe did not remember how he had got here. Throughout the 10 years he had been living on the streets he had been so careful not to put himself at risk of injury. He knew that the streets were a dangerous place to be at times and that his health generally was going downhill, but he hated hospitals with a passion.

His wife had died in hospital and although he had visited her frequently at the time, he could not get over the feeling of powerlessness, and the antiseptic smell made him feel sick.

Joe knew that paramedics had brought him into the hospital trauma centre and that his head hurt. But he had no idea why, or what had happened to him. The nurse who was looking after him had introduced herself as Carol. He looked very carefully, but he could see no sign of judgement in her eyes. He was used to seeing looks of disgust or people looking away when they saw him, so he was an expert at sensing people who looked down on him because he was homeless. They did not understand that once you lost all hope, self-respect and money, there was nowhere else to go. When his wife, Gina, had died from cancer, she was in such pain that he genuinely did not want her distress to continue. But he loved her so much, and she was the only person who had ever believed in him or loved him. His childhood had not been a happy one and when he met Gina he could not believe that anyone as bright and bubbly as her could feel the way she did about him. After she died, he could not cope with work or being with anyone. He lost his home, and living on the streets was his only option.

Carol smiled kindly at him as she explained that he had been attacked and that his head injury was quite serious. Apparently, he needed sutures in the wound and a scan to check for internal bleeding. Carol was obviously very busy, but she kept coming back to see him throughout her shift. When he'd had the scan and his head had been stitched there was no reason for him to stay. Carol seemed concerned about how he would cope after he left, which surprised him. She had made sure that he had antibiotics for the chest infection that she recognised that he had. She also told him that she had seen head lice in his hair and discussed with him what treatment he might find easiest to use. She then used the lotion on his hair that they had discussed and told him to wash it off 12 hours later. She had contacted the night shelter and had arranged a bed for him for the night. He knew that he would be able to have a shower there and wash off the lotion in the morning.

Joe knew that Carol must have stayed on after the end of her shift to arrange these things, and felt deeply touched that she had cared so much about him. She obviously could see past what he looked like and saw the person underneath. This made him feel so much better about himself than he could possibly have imagined.

Discussion

Joe was in a very vulnerable position. He hated hospitals, had unpleasant memories of them, and avoided them at all costs. It would have been very easy for Carol to have cared for his head wound, but not to have become involved with his other health needs. She could have justified this to herself because she was busy and nurses in a trauma centre cannot hope to be holistic in their care, in relation to all potential needs of an individual. They need to address the priorities they are faced with, to minimise risk to all of their patients. It would be easy to see that the multiple and complex needs of a homeless man should be restricted to his major presenting problem: his head wound. However, even if this was the only priority, Joe needed to be treated with respect and compassion. He had been attacked in the street and was in pain, but again it would have been easy for Carol to have not seen past the fact that he was homeless. Joe was very clear that he had been treated with compassion, and this experience might have made him feel less frightened of medical and nursing care in the future.

From Carol's perspective, she felt real compassion for Joe and went out of her way to assess his health needs and work in partnership with him to treat his head lice in a way that fitted in with his lifestyle. She could see beyond the fact that Joe was homeless, to the frightened and vulnerable man in her care. Carol's non-judgemental attitude and her understanding of the fact that we are all different, and that our diversity makes us special, allows us to develop a level of cultural competence, which will be discussed further in Chapter 5. It is easy to be compassionate and caring in some situations, while others stretch our ability more. In a busy trauma centre, a homeless man with a head wound might stretch some nurses' ability to be compassionate to a greater extent, particularly when the person is infested with head lice.

Tweddle (2007), in a Scottish paper, says that 'compassionate care means to actively care. It's about assessing individual needs and it's about the relationships you have with patients. It's much more complex than just being nice to people' (p. 18). Carol clearly demonstrated the fact that she was building a trusting relationship with Joe and she was actively caring for him, in his particular situation. In a Norwegian study, Hem and Heggen (2004) say that 'a compassionate person acts without thought of reward' (p. 22). Carol did just this and, in fact, stayed on after the end of her shift to arrange a night shelter for Joe. All her actions and attitudes demonstrate clearly her compassionate care for him.

Compassion is viewed differently in different faiths. For example, in the Buddhist faith, compassion is referred to as karuna. The aim is perceived to be to relieve the suffering of others by embracing those in distress with a genuine desire to keep them from further harm. Carol was trying to protect Joe from further harm in his vulnerable state. However, it is also seen in the

Buddhist faith as important to have compassion for ourselves in order to feel compassion towards others. This concept of compassion is reflected in other religions and is clearly demonstrated in the parable of the Good Samaritan in Christianity, and as rahman or rahim in the Islamic faith. We are not always compassionate towards ourselves as nurses, or to our colleagues.

We need to try to ensure that our practice areas demonstrate a compassion for other members of the team who are experiencing problems in their personal or professional lives. However, this is often far from the case. Students in our practice areas should be able to feel comfortable in the fact that they are learning nursing in a caring environment, and this should be evident in nurses' care of other nurses, as well as in the care of their patients.

Joe and Carol's perspectives on what compassion is might well have been very different, but in this case study both their views were similar. It is important to understand what patients and clients understand by compassion, as well as what nurses feel encompasses compassionate care. These two perspectives will now be discussed in greater depth.

What does compassion mean to patients and clients?

CASE STUDY 1.2

Paula was struggling to know what to say to the new patient on her ward. Pete had been admitted at midnight; the ward was quieter now and she could sit with him and try to discuss his situation, rather than just deal with the physical needs he had on admission.

Pete was lying down, facing away from her and he was clearly very distressed. All she knew was that he had attempted to commit suicide by taking a large overdose. On handover from the trauma ward, where Pete had been briefly, the nurse who had accompanied him had just given her a brief résumé of his physical status. The nurse had then made some offhand comment that Paula hoped had not been overheard by Pete, about him being another timewaster. Now Paula wanted to see if Pete chose to share with her the reason for his extreme distress, and why he thought that suicide was the only way out. She had never been of the view that the majority of people who attempted suicide were 'just cries for help'. The very term 'cry for help' indicated to her that there was serious distress and yet nurses seemed to minimise this and regard it as attention seeking, rather than a genuine need for help.

Paula gently asked him why he was so unhappy. Pete responded that he could not succeed in anything in life – even his plan to end his own life had been unsuccessful. He told her that he had recently broken up with his long-term girlfriend, who had left him soon after he had been made redundant from his highly paid job in finance. He did not know if these two events were linked, but the extent of his desperation was clear. He had lost his work identity, status and income and then his relationship with the person he considered to be his life partner had ended with a text message saying that she had found someone else.

Pete had moved in with a friend, who had agreed to a house-share as he was struggling to pay the mortgage, and Pete was not coping with his own mortgage repayments since losing his job. Pete had been planning his suicide for a few weeks now and when his friend planned to go away for the weekend he thought that the timing would be perfect. His friend was leaving straight from work on Friday evening and returning straight to work on Monday morning and not coming home again until the evening. Pete had waited until after his friend would have left for his weekend, just in case he came home unexpectedly after finishing work. He then took his planned overdose and was only dimly aware of his housemate returning unexpectedly on the Friday evening and calling the paramedics.

Paula could see how Pete would feel that he could not even succeed with his suicide, despite planning it meticulously. This would have made his sense of failure feel worse. Then, on arrival at the hospital, he was treated as if he had just been attention seeking and not actually being serious in his attempt to die. Paula held his shoulder as he wept and tried to communicate to him that she could understand his feelings of distress and failure at how tonight had turned out for him.

Discussion

Pete was in a highly distressed state and deeply in need of compassionate nursing care. He might not have been able to define what compassion was, or what aspects of Paula's approach exemplified compassion for him, but he knew when compassion was lacking. His experience on admission to the hospital, and comments made to Paula in his hearing about him being a timewaster, would have significantly added to his emotional distress. The term 'cry for help' is used in a derogatory way in relation to suicide and parasuicide. Paula is right to question the fact that a cry for help is actually that, even if the intent to die was not fully thought through or was used as a means to convey distress to others. However, Pete had genuinely meant to die, and had planned his death meticulously. The fact that he had failed in this, too, was not lost on Paula and her compassion during this case study was clearly evident. It is possible that she might have gone a small way towards renewing his faith in humanity by her approach. Something in his emotional state needed to change in order for him to see life as worthwhile. Otherwise he would make another attempt to end his life, which would probably prove successful, given his level of desperation and his clear wish to die.

It is important to know what patients and clients see as compassionate care. Attree (2001), in a UK study, has researched what patients and relatives perceive as key components of high quality care. Respect for an individual's rights, dignity and privacy, as well as involvement in decision making and being given choices about their care and treatment options are seen as paramount. The importance of choice and involving patients in decision making will be discussed further in Chapters 6 and 7. Staff who are 'friendly, warm, sociable and approachable and who developed a bond or rapport' (Attree 2001, p. 461) were perceived by patients to be 'good' practitioners. Paula clearly demonstrated respect for Pete in his current distress. She did not judge him for his actions and she saw him as a priority in how she could spend her time to best effect during that long night for Pete.

Pete had clear mental health needs and there has been some movement to introduce increased understanding of mental health needs into the curriculum for all nursing students. Ensuring that nursing students listen and do not make assumptions about needs is an important part of compassionate care, whether this is in relation to people with mental health needs or the needs of older people. It is important also to be fully aware of the needs of carers and relatives. Finding Pete in the state he was in would have distressed Pete's housemate, and suicide and parasuicide tends to leave family and friends with immense feelings of guilt. This could be in relation to how supportive they have been, whether they could have missed important signs about the depth of despair the person was feeling or what they could have done to prevent the situation.

Rapaport, *et al.* (2006) discuss the importance of assessing the health needs of carers who were looking after people with mental health needs. This would be important in a situation similar to Pete's, where a friend, relative or carer was very traumatised by knowing that their loved one had felt so desperate – whether they had succeeded in their suicide or not. However, carers – who can be very socially isolated – can have very real mental health needs of their own, and these too can go unrecognised. Every carer had a right to an 'individual carer's assessment of his/her circumstances and wishes in assisting understanding of the care context and enhancing appropriate information sharing between professionals and carers' (p. 357). Relatives or carers of people with mental health problems have criticised professionals for their failure to acknowledge their needs and share information with them.

Allowing patients to express their emotions will influence how they adapt to illness and subsequent lifestyle changes (Bowman 2001). Paula clearly gave Pete the opportunity to discuss his emotions that night and anybody suffering from a change in their health status should have the same opportunities. Their health might have deteriorated to the point where life is intolerable, in the same way as Pete's emotional state had brought him to that point. Giving someone the opportunity to discuss their feelings and emotions is an essential part of compassionate care, as is a comprehensive holistic assessment to determine their coping strategies (Loeb 2006).

A lack of compassion has also been highlighted as a problem for people in care homes. This lack of focus on emotional care can make the difference between life being manageable or intolerable for an individual. Using the name they wish to be called by and using appropriate touch and eye contact is essential, as is taking the time to listen to their personal story. The five-foot space around the bed is your whole world if you are confined to bed and it really matters what comes into that space. Fear of old age and death can cause contempt, dehumanisation and potential abuse as well as a lack of empathy and compassion in some nurses. Pete was a victim of this dehumanisation in the trauma ward. Maybe we do not want to think that we could ever become desperate enough to want to commit suicide, or that we will become old, vulnerable and unwanted, so we distance ourselves and this results in a lack of compassion. Society's attitudes, and the culture of care services moving towards targets and away from therapeutic touch and empathetic care, can also be a factor in our less compassionate healthcare services. Our health services are creaking, resources are sparse and the needs of those who have multiple care needs or who are older can be a lower priority than those we can cure. Nurses need to be able to look at who an older person is and what lies beneath the outer image, to the person who still feels young, but who is trapped in an older body. Older people want to be treated well, and as individuals and live their lives to the full. There might need to be more education and training in nursing to reduce the fear of death and ageing as well as increase interpersonal skills and compassion in nursing.

Loneliness, boredom and helplessness epitomise the lives of many people who live among us. This is a distressing thought and one that we might feel we want to distance ourselves from, but this is not possible if we are to retain our humanity, empathy and compassion.

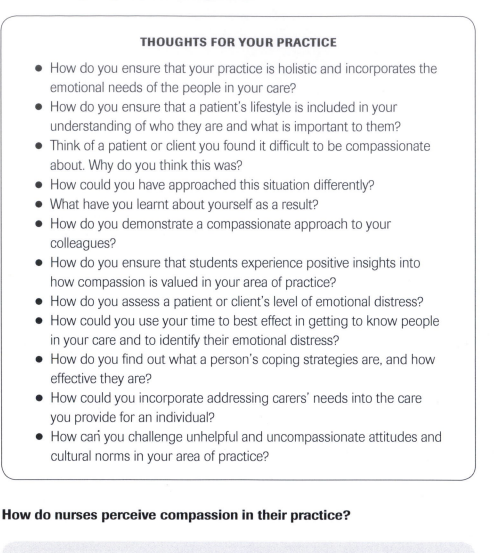

THOUGHTS FOR YOUR PRACTICE

- How do you ensure that your practice is holistic and incorporates the emotional needs of the people in your care?
- How do you ensure that a patient's lifestyle is included in your understanding of who they are and what is important to them?
- Think of a patient or client you found it difficult to be compassionate about. Why do you think this was?
- How could you have approached this situation differently?
- What have you learnt about yourself as a result?
- How do you demonstrate a compassionate approach to your colleagues?
- How do you ensure that students experience positive insights into how compassion is valued in your area of practice?
- How do you assess a patient or client's level of emotional distress?
- How could you use your time to best effect in getting to know people in your care and to identify their emotional distress?
- How do you find out what a person's coping strategies are, and how effective they are?
- How could you incorporate addressing carers' needs into the care you provide for an individual?
- How can you challenge unhelpful and uncompassionate attitudes and cultural norms in your area of practice?

How do nurses perceive compassion in their practice?

CASE STUDY 1.3

Sarah had been visiting Kusumam for some months and she felt desperately sorry for her. As a public health nurse, Sarah was used to home and personal circumstances that were distressing, and she felt desperately sorry for people who had to live their lives in certain ways. However, Kusumam's situation was ongoing and Sarah felt that it would be difficult for her situation to change.

Kusumam and Tom had been living in the area for six months, and they had met when he was working in India. Apparently he had been very sociable, friendly and loving when they had first been together in India. The problems had started when she had returned with him to his home country. He had been increasingly stressed and was very controlling with her. She was not allowed to spend any money and he constantly criticised her for everything from the odd piece of washing left out to dry, or one of the baby's toys left out when he got home, to the general state of their immaculate home. His criticism of Kusumam was very hurtful. He said he found her unattractive, would not let her wear make-up and would not let her learn English or go out.

Kusumam had been learning English without Tom knowing because she wanted to communicate with others when she went out, which she was not able to do very often. Within a few weeks of living here, he had started physically attacking her and forcing himself on her sexually when she was pregnant, but he was careful not to leave her with bruises in obvious places. Kusumam had found the courage to tell Sarah when she visited her, after the baby was born, and the violence was clearly escalating. Tom was besotted with his son and from what Kusumam said, Sarah had no concern for the boy's safety. However, she was deeply concerned for Kusumam's physical and emotional health.

Kusumam had said how much it helped talking to Sarah and that she felt she genuinely understood her situation. She was so far away from her home country and had no money to return there. Her parents did not have the money to help her return either. Sarah understood why she was progressively losing confidence and how fearful she was. Sarah also knew that, for Kusumam's own safety, she needed to escape from Tom's controlling and abusive behaviour. Kusumam felt powerless to do this and embarrassed about how she had got into this situation. She felt that everyone in both their families would blame her if she left and would not believe her side of the story.

So Sarah carried on visiting Kusumam, or seeing her at the health centre. She hoped that the fact that she understood why Kusumam felt unable to leave and take control of her life, and the fact that she was genuinely concerned for her, would gradually help her to gain the confidence she needed to leave her home for good. They had discussed possible strategies for her to use if she were ever to leave, and strategies to try to keep herself as safe as possible, but only Kusumam could make that vital decision to leave.

Discussion

Kusumam clearly felt that Sarah demonstrated compassion towards her in her current situation. It can be difficult for others outside the situation, where they see women living with controlling and abusive men, to comprehend why they choose to stay. They cannot understand that it is not a real choice in most situations. Even the most assertive people feel oppressed by constant rejection, intimidation and violence. If we were in this situation, it would so severely affect our self-esteem that we would be unlikely to be able to find the confidence to leave. For someone like Kusumam who has nowhere else to go, is a long way from their home country and does not understand what help is available, this would feel impossible. Men who suffer abuse from their female or male partners would find it difficult to admit that they are unable to defend themselves or cope with the emotional abuse they are suffering. Women who are living with well-respected men who are influential or have incomes that allow them to be in a good financial situation might find it hard to see that others would believe anything negative about their partner. They might also feel that it might disadvantage their children if they left their affluent situation, or that they would lose their children because they might choose to stay with their father. In addition to this, men and women in this situation can feel that it would be impossible for anyone else to love them and yet they can continue to feel great love for their partner and make excuses for their behaviour.

Therefore, practitioners, like Sarah in her public health nursing role, or trauma centre nurses, could easily think that the solution was simple: just leave the abusive partner. Perhaps we have been lucky enough not to have found ourselves in this situation, and believe that we would be able to deal with such a situation in a more assertive manner. This attitude would stand in the way of being compassionate to someone in Kusumam's situation. Morse, *et al.* (2006) in an American study, says that:

> Compassion is a strong emotion or sentiment stimulated by the presence of suffering that evokes recognition and mutual sharing of the despair or pain of the sufferer. It demonstrates acceptance of the sufferer's plight. But rather than being an expression of the care giver's sorrow (as in sympathy), the compassionate care giver echoes the sufferer's sentiment and shares in the suffering. In sharing the other's suffering, the care giver expresses compassion that strengthens and comforts the sufferer. (p. 80)

This is what Sarah has managed to do. She can share in Kusumam's suffering, despite having never been in a similar situation herself. Through her compassionate approach, Sarah can give strength and comfort to Kusumam and accept that at this moment in time Kusumam has not got the strength to leave her husband.

It would be possible for Sarah to want to distance herself from Kusumam's situation. After all, we like to think that some horrible situation would never happen to us, and if we meet someone who seems to have similarities to us we identify with them more and can feel their suffering more strongly. This can cause difficulties to us, as nurses, because confronting our own mortality and suffering can be 'even worse than death' (Copp cited in Morse 2006, p. 80). It is not possible to avoid pain and still be compassionate; therefore, nurses can withdraw or shield themselves from the suffering of others, which is the antithesis of compassion.

A joint primary care trust (PCT) and university initiative in Scotland uses the nursing curriculum within the university to try to develop compassion among student nurses (Tweddle 2007, citing Lothian PCT and Napier University). They use a Compassionate Care Project to understand, identify and showcase areas of good practice in compassionate care to disseminate knowledge and enhance practice elsewhere. This is integrated into the undergraduate nursing programme to help nurses engage and build on relationships with their patients in order to gain a greater understanding of what compassion means in their practice.

THOUGHTS FOR YOUR PRACTICE

- Think of a patient or client who you felt compassionate for because of the way they had to lead their lives.
- How did you share in this patient or client's 'suffering'?
- How did your actions strengthen or comfort your patient or client?
- What have you learnt about yourself from this experience for your future practice?
- Can you think of someone you found it hard to be compassionate towards?
- Why do you think this was the case?
- Try to think of ways in which you could have increased your level of compassion in this situation.
- Do you find it easy to share your patients' suffering? If not why do you think this could be the case?

KEY THEME TWO – CARING

CASE STUDY 1.4

Brenda did not want to be here. She had been in hospital several times before, but it had never felt like this. Last time she was in this ward, admittedly, standards seemed to have slipped, but she thought that they were just understaffed at the time. In the past she had felt safe here and that there were caring people who understood her and what she needed. She felt that it genuinely mattered to the nursing staff whether she was in pain or uncomfortable.

This time Brenda had been very upset by what she had seen. Nurses seemed to be avoiding eye contact with all the patients. Even when they were with a patient they appeared to be doing what needed to be done at the time, but they did not seem to be making an effort to talk to them. Brenda heard one nurse, who had been asked a simple question by a patient, turn to her with a glare and say, 'What do you want?', before she stormed off. The nurse had only just come on duty and the lady who asked the question was in her eighties. Brenda would never forget the look of embarrassment and humiliation as the lady turned away with tears in her eyes. When they were rude and brusque to Brenda she had felt hurt and dismissed, but it was far worse to see it happening to a frail, vulnerable old lady.

The student nurses were actually very caring, but when Brenda saw how rude the qualified nurses were, she wondered how long the students would stay like that. Would they too think that it was all right to treat people with such disdain? Brenda had seen people being ignored when they were calling for help. She had seen people crying in pain when their calls for pain relief were ignored. She had seen people being left in the toilet stranded as they could not get back on their own. Call bells were left ringing for a long time and she heard a nurse say, 'I am going to fill my care plans in here, because they keep insisting on ringing their bells and I am sick of going to them to help.' Brenda had also seen nurses chatting at the nurses' station and had overheard a sister saying very delicate and private things about patients to each other in front of her and other patients.

Brenda wanted to go home, although she knew she was not well enough. Nurses were meant to care, weren't they? They should not go into a caring profession if they did not care.

Discussion

The patient in this case study clearly felt that her needs were not being met, but she felt even worse for the older and more vulnerable people who were being treated with rudeness and a lack of caring and compassion. She rightly questioned why people come into nursing if they do not care. Defining what caring actually is can be difficult, although we use the word all the time in relation to our practice; for example: nursing care, social care, care environment, caregiver and care assistant. So what does it actually mean? Again, it often can be understood more from situations where it is lacking, rather than from where it exists.

Watson (1988), an American academic who has extensively analysed the nature of caring, suggests that although there is no consensus about the definition of caring, there are common aspects. Watson says that caring involves wanting to care, intending to care, and actions that are caring by nature. It is clear from this case study that the nurses involved did not seem to want to care or intend to care and are therefore not translated into caring actions. The patient in the case study rightly questions whether the students on the ward, who appear more caring, might become negatively influenced by this negative attitude towards caring or lack of caring.

The following five themes are proposed by Swanson (1991) in relation to caring: knowing, being with, doing for, enabling, and maintaining belief. Other discussions of contemporary caring in healthcare include such terms as interest and concern, liking, giving care, compassion, and commitment (Kim-Godwin, *et al.* 2001). The nurses on the ward in the case study do not appear to want to spend time with their patients, even when they are less busy. They also are rude, do not maintain confidentiality and actively humiliate patients in their care. We would suggest that if these nurses wanted to show the fact that they cared for their patients they would be:

➤ getting to know their patients;
➤ showing interest in them;
➤ liking, valuing and respecting them as people;
➤ wanting to spend time with them;
➤ wanting to ease their suffering by doing things for them;
➤ increasing their self-esteem and self-belief;
➤ empowering them to feel more in control;
➤ showing concern for them;
➤ being committed to giving them high quality care;
➤ acting in a compassionate manner.

Caring has to be a conscious act, according to Watson (1999). She identifies several themes in relation to caring in nursing:
➤ connection to the individual;
➤ relationship with the individual;
➤ a caring relationship and caring environment, which are central to promoting human dignity, a sense of identity and integrity;
➤ empowerment, which encourages self-awareness and self-knowledge and which has a positive impact on healing.

In contrast, a UK British Medical Association study (BMA, 2005) of the values doctors perceive to be important in being a good doctor are in the following order: competence, integrity, caring, compassion, responsibility, commitment, advocacy, confidentiality and spirit of enquiry. It is good to see that compassion and caring are listed here as important traits in a doctor. However, referring to this study in an editorial, Godlee (2008) highlights the importance of the values starting with the letter 'C' and says that 'caring sounds like a soft option on the list of values – but it isn't when used in the sense of taking care' (www.bmj.com/cgi/content/full/336/7649/0) and equates it to reducing medical error. While this is very important, it is interesting that this interpretation means that doctors do not necessarily value caring in its own right as a core professional value. Godlee (2008) adds to the 'C' list communication and the ability to say sorry in order to reduce patient complaints, as well as confidentiality, competition (to improve patient care) and concordance. Maybe for doctors for whom curing is a central philosophy, caring is seen as a 'soft' value whereas competence, commitment and avoiding complaints are seen as more important. This is not to say that doctors do not care, but just that other values are seen as more essential.

For nurses, caring has always been seen as an important component of nursing practice and is clearly lacking in the Case study 1.4.

In developing our discussion on the meaning of caring, we feel it is important to consider 'practice wisdom'. Tichen and Higgs (2001) define practice wisdom as 'the possession of practice experience and knowledge together with the ability to use them critically, intuitively and practically. Including characteristics of clarity, discernment and caring deeply from an objective stance, practice wisdom is a component of professional artistry' (p. 275). The Royal College of Nursing (RCN) (2005, p. 23) say that the attributes of practice wisdom include:
➤ holistic practice knowledge, including using all forms of knowledge in practice;

➤ saliency, including active listening, picking up on cues and responding to needs;

➤ knowing the patient, including having respect for people and their view of the world;

➤ moral agency, which includes promoting dignity and respecting their individuality;

➤ skilled know-how, which involves problem solving and responding to individual situations.

All these components of practice wisdom are essential, but we would like to see more of an emphasis on compassion and caring. A nurse can actively listen to a patient or client, promote their dignity and show respect for them and still fail to show that they care for them as a person.

As a Greek study carried out by Rovithis and Parissopoulos (2005) says:

> Intuition in practice has been linked to enhanced clinical judgement, effective decision making and crisis aversion . . . if intuition is ignored practitioners will become entrenched in standardised procedures and routines of care and there will be little opportunity for the flair and skill of nursing judgement to flourish (p. 6).

Intuition is part of the art of nursing, which we discuss further in Chapter 2 in relation to sensitivity.

We believe that intuitive and sensitive practice are essential components of caring in nursing and agree with the view expressed in Case study 1.4, that if this is missing, nurses become task orientated and standardised in their approach to patients, which is the antithesis of caring.

Therefore, we now intend to focus on what caring actually means in nursing practice and how we build caring relationships with our patients and clients.

Do we understand the importance of caring in nursing practice?

CASE STUDY 1.5

Ian had been in hospital many times over his short life. He was now 14 years old and his cystic fibrosis had resulted in another stay in hospital. He had visited his grandfather on the male medical ward in this same hospital and knew that he would not want to be admitted there. The ward seemed to be full of men who seemed very old and who seemed to have serious symptoms and horrible coughs.

However, Ian was starting to feel that he was outgrowing the children's ward. When he was younger, he enjoyed the company of other children and once he started to feel a little better it was usually a fun place to be. Now, though, he was older and he knew that his body was changing and doing strange things that he did not always understand. When younger children burst into the bathroom or appeared behind his screens he was embarrassed and he was finding the lack of privacy a real problem this time. On top of that, all the activities available on the ward were designed for much younger children and he was bored. His mother had promised to bring him his MP3 player, but his computer-based games were not going to be a possibility.

He had been speaking to Sheila, one of the nurses on the ward, and she seemed to understand how he felt. She was always very careful to totally close the screens around his bed so that there were no gaps that people could see through. She explained that they were campaigning to change the ward so that there was a separate section for young people. She had asked him what would help his stay in hospital to be more comfortable and she had requested that the play specialist, Maria, come and see him. He had felt that the very name 'play specialist' meant that she would not understand his interests – after all, he did not see what he did in his leisure time as 'play'. He was wrong, though, because Maria said that making sure that he was stimulated was part of his recovery and she found a laptop from somewhere and gave him some computer games that he really enjoyed. Ian was very pleased that he had discussed his worries with Sheila, because now he could see that the other nurses were making sure that his privacy was maintained and that the younger children did not bother him when he felt unwell. At other times he was more than happy to talk and play with them and show them how to get better at the games they were playing. He just could not cope with it all the time and sometimes he felt so exhausted. At those times, there always seemed to be someone who would notice his tiredness and distract the other children away from him so he could rest.

Discussion

Ian felt very vulnerable in this child-centred environment, although, as he said, the transition to an adult ward would prove even more difficult for him. This transition to adult services from children's services is not easy for young people to cope with. More and more children with life-limiting and life-threatening illnesses are surviving into adulthood. Having to make the transition to adult services can be traumatic, with different medical and nursing staff and different wards, all of which can feel less personal.

Sheila and Maria recognised the fact that Ian's needs were different to those of the younger children and made every effort to understand those needs, which are related to his total care, rather than the treatment he requires. Watson (2000) makes the point that 'caring as a relationship cannot be reduced to a hierarchy of tasks and skills that one "does"' (p. 8). Sheila could have carried out the 'curing' or treatment part of her role, through a series of nursing tasks, without really understanding some of the factors that were negatively impacting on the 'caring' that was part of Ian's recovery. The relationship between Ian and Sheila and her colleagues was an essential part of this caring. Caring is perceived by Watson (2000) to be creating a situation where someone can express their vulnerability, which is part of being human. Watson says that 'if we are not able to be vulnerable with ourselves and others, we become robotic, mechanical, detached and depersonal in our lives and work and relationships' (p. 8). This ability to be vulnerable with others and ourselves is part of being self-aware and empathetic, which will be discussed further in Chapter 2. We need to be in touch with who we are, even in the midst of illness; this can be seen in Ian and Sheila both recognising what is important for Ian's identity and recovery.

The Department of Health in the UK have issued some best practice guidelines in relation to caring. These guidelines, called Confidence in Caring (DOH 2008), were based on feedback from patients about what is important to them. The patients were from acute hospital environments, but their points are valid for all care environments. If nurses 'care for' patients, but do not 'care about' them (p. 5), then they are again able to carry out mechanistic tasks, but without necessarily seeing the person as a whole. If this is the case, can nurses really believe that they are carrying out the caring and compassionate part of their role? Sheila was clearly caring for and about Ian in trying to solve some of the issues that he had in relation to his care and care environment.

Nursing care is becoming more and more complex and the person behind the health condition or health need can be easily lost. A nurse has to practise the art as well as the science of her nursing role, and this will again be discussed in Chapter 2. In this case, Sheila's sensitivity and empathy were part of the art of her nursing practice. In the Confidence in Caring guidelines (DOH 2008), patients talked about the importance of the care environment and how the nursing team interacted with one another, as well as patients and their relatives. This becomes part of the culture of the care environment, which we have discussed already in this chapter. It will be discussed again in Chapter 3, including how nurses can become 'acculturalised' within their practice base to what is considered to be the norm for practice. This can be a positive or negative culture, which can encourage caring and compassion, or perceive these as less important aspects of the nursing role. We believe, in this case, that this negative perception of the importance of caring and compassion would be just about treating a patient, rather than truly caring for them. In such an environment, staff would not feel confident to exhibit caring traits and, therefore, this confidence to care would not be passed on to their patients or clients. For example, if a trauma centre has a negative culture in relation to those who self-harm or attempt suicide, then this culture would make it difficult for individual nurses to be empathetic or use therapeutic touch, as discussed further in Chapters 2 and 4. What are we then teaching our students and future practitioners about the importance of care within our nursing roles?

Patients in the Confidence in Caring guidelines (DOH 2008) say that how nurses behave and look, as well as how they talk to people, is as important as what they actually say. We have to remember that in some traumatic situations where a loved one is very ill, dying, or has already died, their friends and family might remember what we say, and the way we say it, for the rest of their lives. This is an immense responsibility that we need to take very seriously. For us it is just another busy shift, for them it is a time when their lives changed forever. Patients and clients have a right to be treated with kindness and courtesy at all times, but caring and compassion go beyond this to reveal more about our basic humanity and care for others. People do not want to hear about staffing or team issues or our personal lives when they are feeling ill and frightened; our focus should be totally on them. They might not question our professional competence and expertise, but they might have less confidence about how much they feel cared about when they are in a vulnerable situation. Sheila clearly demonstrated to Ian that she understood why privacy and an appropriately stimulating environment were important to him, and were essential parts of his nursing care.

The Confidence in Caring guidelines (DOH 2008, p. 6) say that the factors that create confidence in care are:

➤ a calm, clean, safe environment;
➤ a positive friendly culture;
➤ good team working and good relationships;
➤ well-managed care with efficient delivery;
➤ personalised care for and about every patient.

Patients say that what they want from healthcare providers are (DOH 2008, p. 28):

➤ a care provider who looks and behaves professionally; is caring, competent, knowledgeable and compassionate and provides holistic, timely, seamless care and information;

➤ a care partner who works with patients and relatives to plan care, gives constant feedback and reports, and helps them to navigate the health and social care system;

➤ a champion who puts their interests first and protects them when they are vulnerable;

➤ a coordinator who is constant, accessible and accountable for communicating the plan and monitoring the delivery of care.

The DOH guidelines give very helpful pointers about what patients want from nurses and the care environment. We have written this whole book from the perspective of patients and clients and how things appear to them, and what exemplifies caring and compassionate practice.

THOUGHTS FOR YOUR PRACTICE

- How is caring viewed in your practice area?
- How does this influence your practice and that of others?
- Do you think that there are times when you focus more on the tasks to be carried out rather than the person?
- What sorts of situations cause this to happen?
- Can you think of any ways in which you can enhance your focus on the person at these times?
- Can you think of ways in which you can help students to understand this important emphasis within practice?
- Do you sometimes feel that although you 'care for' your patients or clients that you are not always able to 'care about' them? If so how could you enhance this in your practice?
- Do you think that you could sometimes focus more on your caring relationships with patients and clients? If so, how?
- Think of examples where you focus on caring as well as curing in your nursing care.
- Can you think of how you can increase the caring aspects, even when curing has to be the central focus of your interventions?

- Do you feel that you need to start to question the culture of your practice environment, in terms of how caring it is?
- If so, how can you start to encourage discussion about this with your colleagues?
- If not, how can you use your caring culture as an exemplar for others and for students who come to your practice area?
- Consider the role of 'care provider'; are there any aspects of the role that you could enhance?
- Consider the role of 'care partner'; are there any aspects of the role that you could enhance?
- Consider the role of 'champion'; are there any aspects of the role that you could enhance?
- Consider the role of 'coordinator'; are there any aspects of the role that you could enhance?

How do we build caring relationships with individuals?

CASE STUDY 1.6

Mabel had been sitting looking out of the window waiting for Richard. She did so enjoy his visits to dress her leg. He always made her laugh and was very sensitive in his understanding of what it might feel like to be totally housebound. Her neighbour popped in occasionally, but she was an only child so she had no living relatives following the death of her husband Bert. Mabel's friends had died before her and really there was nobody to care about her at all. She dreaded the time when her leg had healed and Richard stopped visiting. Who would know if she was ill and who would find her when she died?

Richard was very aware of Mabel's social isolation and was very concerned about her. She was unable to go out and had been so close to Bert that they had never really needed anyone else in their lives. Richard could see how Mabel had deteriorated since her husband's death and she had told him that she was not afraid of dying because she knew that she would be reunited with her beloved Bert. She was worried about being alone or dying without anybody there and she did not want to be one of those people whose body was found weeks after their death.

Richard's priorities in visiting Mabel were far more than dressing her leg ulcer. His caring nature meant that he would really like her to be somewhere where she felt cared for. She had such a strong sense of humour and he was sure she would be popular wherever she went. She loved the company of others and was in the process of selling her house, which was cold and damp, in order to move into a residential home. This decision had not been made lightly, but Richard and Mabel had discussed it at length and Mabel was confident in the decision she had made. Richard was very fond of Mabel and thought of his elderly Aunt Rene, who he was very close to. How would she manage in Mabel's situation? He felt pleased that Mabel had wanted to share her feelings on how life felt for her. He was very careful not to try to influence her decision, but knew that she needed more information in order to feel happy about where she would end up living. He could see how much more positive she was feeling just knowing that she had made the decision to sell her home. He had ideas for possible agencies to get involved if Mabel's ulcer healed before her move took place and he was discussing options with her. Mabel had already agreed to meet people who could come and visit her at home, and that was a good start.

Discussion

Mabel had very real, undisputed and measurable needs in relation to her leg ulcer that were the reason for Richard's visits. There was no reason to doubt the need for visits to help her wound to heal and success could be measured by how quickly the ulcer healed. However, some needs are less predictable and can be disputed by others; therefore they are less measurable (Health Visitor Association [HVA] 1995). In Mabel's case, her social isolation, loneliness and fears about being ill or dying on her own are not the reason for Richard's visits, but they are part of holistic and compassionate care. In the present day, outcome-based and more measurable needs are clearly prioritised in a resource deprived health service. However, if these needs are the only priorities then our nursing care will inevitably become less about caring and more about curing, as already discussed. Nursing should continue to incorporate the less predicted needs of patients, such as hidden social and emotional needs, in order to keep a central focus on care. These could include the effects of poverty and local crime rates that make individuals feel threatened. In Mabel's situation, these would include her bereavement, loneliness, social isolation, poverty, inability to access services due to being housebound and lack of transport. These types of need are often much higher priorities for patients and clients than the fact that they have a leg ulcer, or whatever else necessitates a nurse's involvement. If they do not feel that the nurse is interested in the things that worry them most, they do not feel that the nurse cares and a therapeutic relationship cannot develop.

Watson (1985) discusses this development of a therapeutic relationship, and says that this relies on 10 carative factors:

➤ the formation of a humanistic and altruistic system of values where the nurse uses their sense of humanity and their caring about others;
➤ the instillation of faith or hope;
➤ cultivation of sensitivity to one's self and to others, which incorporates self-awareness and empathy;
➤ development of a helping and trusting relationship;
➤ encouraging and accepting expression of positive and negative feelings;
➤ the systematic use of scientific problem-solving method for decision making;
➤ promotion of interpersonal teaching and learning;
➤ provision of a supportive, protective or empowering emotional, physical, socio-cultural, and spiritual environment;
➤ assisting with meeting the needs of the individual;
➤ the effect of how people view their lives, their coping strategies and what motivates them.

Richard had this relationship with Mabel. He knew what was important to her and what frightened her. He knew how much she missed her husband and how lonely she was. He genuinely cared about her and was trying to help her to feel more hopeful about her future. He was self-aware and knew that it would be easy to take over in terms of problem solving and decision making, and knew how important it was for her to make her own decisions about her future. However, he made sure that he created an environment where she could benefit from his expertise and knowledge of other services available, and could express her fears and what she wanted in her future life. All of these epitomise a therapeutic relationship and holistic care – topics which will be discussed further in Chapters 3 and 7.

> The sensitivity of the nurse in an interpersonal communication encounter is one of the most crucial therapeutic tools for delivering care. Of all the problems that can arise in nursing care, perhaps the most common is failure to establish rapport and a helping–trust relationship with the other person. (Watson 1985, p. 25)

Watson stresses the importance of communicating the fact that the nurse genuinely cares, and getting to know the person in creating an environment where the person can discuss sensitive issues and feelings. This involves being totally focused on the person at that moment in time, which Watson refers to as 'relational caring' (Watson 2000, p. 6). It is important for nurses to try to understand their patient or client as an individual person with different feelings and priorities, rather than as an object of care that can be manipulated or treated the same as everyone else. Nurses need to be genuine, empathetic and self-aware in order to provide high quality care involving real caring in their practice.

'Non-possessive warmth' is also discussed by Watson (1985) – the importance of which is similar to unconditional regard. The nurse's attitude has to be accepting of who the patient is as a person and should be non-judgemental in that acceptance, which will be discussed further in Chapter 5. This needs to be communicated through a nurse's physical care and their verbal and non-verbal communication.

A therapeutic relationship is defined as being '. . . grounded in an interpersonal process that occurs between the nurse and the patient. It is a purposeful, goal-directed relationship that is directed at advancing the best interest and outcome of the patient' (Registered Nurses Association of Ontario [RNAO] cited in Foster and Hawkins 2005, p. 698). The RNAO highlight the importance of active listening, cultural competence, respect, empowerment, self-advocacy and choice in decision making as central to compassionate care. They have designed a knowledge and skills framework, which is aimed at initiating, developing and maintaining effective therapeutic relationships. The knowledge involves an understanding of psychological theories and information gathering, interpersonal and development theory, diversity influences and determinants, the person, their health and illness, broad influences on healthcare and healthcare policy and systems. The skills involve self-knowledge and self-awareness, empathy and respect, observation and listening skills, and awareness of boundaries and referral skills. All of these were again exemplified in Richard's relationship with Mabel and clearly demonstrate his compassionate and caring approach to her and her holistic health needs.

THOUGHTS FOR YOUR PRACTICE

- Think of a patient or client you have been involved with:
  - How did you establish a rapport with them?

> — What helped you to build a helping and trusting relationship with them?
> — In building this relationship what did you learn about yourself that will help you in future practice?
> — What could you pass on to colleagues and students that will help them in their practice?
> - How do you communicate the fact that you care about patients and clients as individuals through your verbal and non-verbal communication?
> - Think of a situation where you felt that you judged a patient or client by their words, actions, behaviour or lifestyle. Can you now think of ways in which you could be less judgemental and more caring in your approach?

SUMMARY – LINKS TO COMPASSION AND CARING

In this chapter we have started to explore some of the very complex issues that surround compassion and care in nursing. We feel passionate about the importance of compassion and genuine care in nursing practice. This has inspired us to try to identify what the central themes are for nurses in carrying out compassionate care. In our opinion, the following themes are essential elements:

➤ empathy and sensitivity;
➤ dignity and respect;
➤ listening and responding;
➤ diversity and cultural competence;
➤ choice and priorities;
➤ empowerment and advocacy.

These themes will form the focus of the chapters in this book. We have used case studies throughout, which are largely from the patient or client's perspective. The reason for this is because, for us, this is the most important perspective if we are to be genuinely compassionate in our care. Our hope is that this approach will help you to build on your current practice and generate ideas that will challenge you to bring about changes in practice for both yourselves and your colleagues. In addition, we hope that this book will help you to teach students in a meaningful way about the importance of compassion and caring in nursing.

REFERENCES

Attree M. Patients' and relatives' experiences and perspectives of 'good' and 'not so good' quality care. *J Adv Nurs.* 2001; **33**(4): 456–66.

Bowman G. Emotions and illness. *J Adv Nurs.* 2001; **34**(2): 256–63.

British Medical Association. *Core Values for the Medical Profession in the 21st Century.* London: BMA; 2005.

Department of Health. *Confidence in Caring: a framework for best practice.* London: Department of Health; 2008.

Foster T, Hawkins J. The therapeutic relationship: dead or merely impeded by technology. *BJN.* 2005; **14**(13): 698–702.

Gadsby A. We need to start seeing the person behind the patient. *Nurs Times.* 2008; **35**: 8.

Godlee F. Editor's choice. *BMJ.* 2008; available at http://bmj.com/cgi/content/full/336/7649/0

Health Visitor Association. *Weights and Measures: outcomes and evaluation in health visiting.* London: Health Visitor Association; 1995.

Hem M, Heggen K. Is compassion central to nursing practice? *Contemp Nurse.* 2004; **17**(1–2): 19–31.

Kim-Godwin Y, Clarke P, Barton L. A model for the delivery of cultural competent community care. *J Adv Nurs.* 2001; **35**(6): 918–25.

Loeb S. African American older adults coping with chronic health conditions. *J Transcult Nurs.* 2006; **17**(2): 139–47.

Morse J, Bottorff J, Anderson G, *et al.* Beyond empathy: expanding expressions of caring. *J Adv Nurs.* 2006; **53**(1): 75–87.

Rapaport J, Bellringer S, Pinfold V, *et al.* Carers and confidentiality in mental healthcare: considering the role of the carer's assessment: a study of service users', carers' and practitioners' views. *Health Soc Care Comm.* 2006; **14**(4): 357–65.

Rovithis M, Parissopoulos S. Intuition in nursing practice. *ICUS Nurs Web J.* 2005; **22**: 1–10.

Royal College of Nursing. *Changing Patients' Worlds Through Nursing Practice Expertise.* London: Royal College of Nursing; 2005.

Swanson K. Empirical development of middle range theory of caring. *Nurs Res.* 1991; **40**(3): 161–6.

Tichen A, Higgs J. Towards professional artistry and creativity in practice. In: Higgs J, Tichen A, editors. *Professional Practice in Health Education and the Creative Arts.* Oxford: Blackwell Science; 2001.

Tweddle L. Compassion on the curriculum. *Nurs Times.* 2007; **103**(38): 18–19.

Watson J. *Nursing: the philosophy and science of caring.* Boulder, CO: University Press of Colorado; 1985.

Watson J. New dimensions of human caring theory. *Nurs Sci Q.* 1988; **1**(4): 175–81.

Watson J. *Postmodern Nursing and Beyond.* Toronto, ON: Churchill Livingstone; 1999.

Watson J. Via negative: considering caring by way of non-caring. *Aust J Holist Nurs.* 2000; **7**(1): 4–8.

Wilkinson C. *Professional Perspectives in Healthcare.* Basingstoke: Palgrave MacMillan; 2007.

www.bma.org.uk/ap.nsf/Content/profval~values

CHAPTER 2

Empathy and sensitivity

Overview of the chapter

Key theme one – empathy
- Case study
- Discussion
- Do we know ourselves, and how do we identify and engage with others?
- Case study
- Discussion
- Thoughts for your practice
- How can we become more emotionally intelligent and can we become emotionally brilliant?
- Case study
- Discussion
- Thoughts for your practice

Key theme two – sensitivity
- Case study
- Discussion
- Do we understand the importance of emotional comfort and the appropriate use of humour?
- Case study
- Discussion
- Thoughts for your practice
- Sensitive care and resources – is there a conflict?
- Case study
- Discussion
- Thoughts for your practice
- Summary – links to compassion and caring
- References

OVERVIEW OF THE CHAPTER

Empathy and sensitivity are key aspects of compassionate nursing care, yet they are often not prioritised or valued within nurse education or the delivery of healthcare. In terms of nursing, it is important to understand what empathy and sensitivity really mean. This chapter aims to help you to consider different parts of these key aspects of compassionate practice, in order to help you to reflect on your current role and develop your future practice.

It is essential to know ourselves and develop our self-awareness, as far as possible, in order to really understand how others feel. Being self-aware is the only way we can become truly empathetic; then we can start to use all the skills of emotional intelligence. However, as nurses, we need to aim for more than just emotional intelligence but strive for 'emotional brilliance' (Goleman 1996). We need to identify more with people in order for them to feel able to engage with us as healthcare practitioners.

Sensitivity needs to be used in addition to empathy to help us promote emotional comfort. Nurses need to capitalise on the art of nursing, as well as the scientific base, in order to deliver holistic care. Humour can be used therapeutically – if used appropriately. Nurses can feel that their moral responsibility towards the patient is being compromised in these financially driven times, and they can feel distressed by the gaps in provision. They can also feel that they have not got the time to truly care or provide quality of care, which can also be distressing. The conflict between providing sensitive care and meeting financial targets can mean that nurses can become desensitised and acculturalised to poor standards of nursing care, as discussed in Chapter 1. These standards are often far below those they would normally aspire to under other circumstances.

All these aspects of empathy and sensitivity will be discussed in this chapter.

KEY THEME ONE – EMPATHY

CASE STUDY 2.1

Judy came into the practice nurse's room with some trepidation. The last time she had been to the surgery was just after the death of her mother. She had been to see the doctor because she just could not seem to sleep at night, or come to terms with the fact that her mother had died so suddenly, or so young. The doctor, who she had not seen before, was so kind and had seemed to understand how devastated she was. She realised that this was the same consulting room, and all the feelings of distress, which were never far from the surface, came back to her with a vengeance. The doctor had suggested that she come back and have her blood pressure checked, as it had been a little high when he measured it. So here she was a month a later, in the same room, feeling the same feelings as she had when she was here before.

The nurse had her back to her and was frowning at the computer screen. She muttered a quick 'sit down' and continued to stare at the screen. Judy sat in the only chair available, which was at right angles to the nurse, who still did not look up. Finally, she introduced herself as Marion and said that she would be with her in a moment, but the computer was playing up. Judy sat still, waiting, but feeling more anxious all the time. This was made worse by the fact that she wanted her blood pressure reading to be low because she really didn't want to start taking tablets. She took deep breaths and looked around the room. All the notices seemed to be about what she shouldn't do ... contact the practice without good reason, be rude to members of staff, fail to cancel appointments that she couldn't come to etc, etc. She could feel her anxiety levels rising and she'd had a couple of panic attacks in the past month or so. She really hoped that she could hold it all together now.

Marion had recently come to the practice from a hospital environment. She really did not like computers very much – they seemed to be aware of this and things tended to go wrong when she used them. She had felt that the paperwork got in the way of her relationship with patients, at times, when she was on the day case ward. There seemed so much to ask, and so many boxes to fill in, with so little time to take a history of the patient's health status before the surgery was to take place. She had moved to a primary care setting, hoping for more long-term relationships with patients. Now she had to cope with the same sort of questions, but using the dreaded computer. She sighed and explained to Judy that she just needed to ask some quick questions about her health before she took her blood pressure and discussed possible ways forward. She started with the family history questions and without looking up asked if her parents were alive and well. Judy answered in a quiet voice that her father was well and had no health problems. Then there was silence.

'And your mother?' Marion asked quickly, wanting to move onto other questions, conscious that she might be starting to run late in her appointments' schedule. She heard a sob and out of the corner of her eye saw Judy stand up. She looked up and was shocked to see tears running down Judy's face and a panicked look on her face. The next thing she knew was that Judy had run from the room, saying she couldn't stay any longer and would make another appointment. Marion had absolutely no idea of what had just happened or why Judy was distressed and felt that she must have done something to upset her, but couldn't begin to understand what.

Discussion

It is clear from the case study that Marion was unable to deliver empathetic and sensitive care. It was not that she did not want to focus on Judy's needs, but she was unable to relate to Judy's situation, or respond to her feelings, because she was so preoccupied and focused on the tools and tasks generated through the computerised assessment process. Moore (2006) says, 'if the clinician is in a bad mood, this may put the client in a bad mood as well; essentially, it is like looking into a mirror'(p. 16). In Judy's case, it was not the fact that Marion was necessarily in a bad mood that was the issue. However, Marion did sigh and frown during the brief time they had together, which could have been seen as her being in a bad mood. Judy consequently felt that she was not interested in her, and possibly that she was causing a problem by just being there. She was then highly unlikely to want to tell her sensitive information that was distressing for her to talk about. As nurses, we need to be aware that if we seem tired, bored, uninterested, tense or in a rush then this will have a negative effect on the relationship with patients. In addition, patients could start to mirror the mood that they think they see in their healthcare practitioner, which cannot fail to affect the amount of information that they are prepared to divulge and the way they view the interaction and nursing care overall.

Moore (2006) goes on to say, 'Imagine how our clients must feel, especially with the additional challenge of a communication disorder, if we are rushed, harried, or curt during our interactions' (p. 17). She then points out that 'Most patients credit their treatment outcome directly to those caregivers who demonstrate a concern for them' (p. 17).

Rungapadiachy (1999) says that 'empathy refers to one's ability to perceive the situation from the other person's point of view' (p. 224). Kirschenbaum and Henderson (1990) say that empathy is 'to sense the client's private world as if it were your own, but without ever losing the "as if" quality' (p. 226). Because Marion was unable to form a relationship with Judy, she was completely unable to sense her discomfort and distress. Empathy does not mean that nurses have to have lived the same lives as their patients, had the same experiences or had the same relationships, but they still need to take time to understand the world as their patient sees it. The dictionary definition says that empathy is 'the ability to imagine oneself in another's place and understand the other's feelings, desires, ideas, and actions' (Britannica Online). McCabe and Timmins (2006) say that 'if nurses fail to empathise with their patients, then they can not help them to understand or cope effectively as individuals with their illness'(p. 72). This was certainly the case in the lack of effective interaction between Marion and Judy.

Moore (2006) quotes an anonymous English author: 'To empathise is to see with the eyes of another, to hear with the ears of another, and to feel with the heart of another' (p. 16), and she suggests that 'the connection between the client and clinician that facilitates a positive influence in treatment is empathy' (p. 16).

It is, perhaps, easier for a nurse aged 25 to understand the devastation of a life-limiting diagnosis and prognosis in a person of their own age. They might find it harder to see that those same feelings exist in someone of 55 or 85, and therefore might not be able to feel that devastation in the same way. The nurse might need to work at developing this degree of empathy by reflecting on other situations they might have known, personally or professionally. As Reynolds and Scott (2000) say, 'The ability to perceive and reason, as well as the ability to communicate understanding of the other person's feelings and their attached meanings is essential in empathetic nursing practice' (p. 226).

In addition, we might want to protect ourselves from the vulnerability of true empathy, as this means that we could see ourselves as being at risk of harm coming to us, or those we love. It is easier to remain a bit detached; in fact, this was taught in the past as a way of coping with traumatic situations in nursing. However, if we can glimpse the 'private world' of our patients, in all its distress, while still keeping the 'as if' quality, we can empathise with them, without feeling submerged and unable to help them. This is the true aim of achieving empathetic care in nursing practice.

Do we know ourselves, and how do we identify and engage with others?

CASE STUDY 2.2

Angie is a midwife who is talking to Tamsin, soon after she has had a miscarriage at 20 weeks' gestation. Angie is genuinely trying to help Tamsin feel more positive about the future. She makes various comments about the fact that at 28 she is still young, there is plenty of time to have other children, plus it would have been far more traumatic if she had lost this child once she was born and that these things often happen for a reason. Tamsin becomes increasingly distressed and angry because she feels that the importance of her loss is being minimised, and that the identity of the daughter that she would have had is not being recognised. Angie's lack of empathy is compounded by her lack of self-awareness. She fails to recognise that her words and thoughts are inappropriate for someone who has just lost a baby. Her words and thoughts might not be untrue, but at this point in time they are totally inappropriate.

Discussion

A key aspect of empathy is getting to know ourselves. Self-awareness can be defined as 'knowing of oneself' (Rungapadiachy 1999, p. 17). He says that self-awareness has three major components:

➤ cognitive – thoughts
➤ affective – feelings
➤ behavioural – actions one takes.

The way people think affects how they feel and, therefore, what they do. Rungapadiachy says that 'if what Freud said is true, that is, people are only aware of roughly 20% of what they say or do, then it does not bear thinking of the potential damage that could be caused when healthcarers interact with clients or patients' (1999, p. 33).

Angie's approach to Tamsin's loss clearly demonstrates the negative impact that a lack of self-awareness can have. Angie's thoughts and feelings about miscarriages at this stage of a pregnancy are influencing what she says to Tamsin and the strategies she tries to use to help Tamsin cope with her loss.

Angie is unable to truly identify with Tamsin's situation as a whole. She is actually reducing Tamsin's distress to the miscarriage alone, without being able to see Tamsin's overall situation. Because she is unable to identify with her, she is therefore unable to have any meaningful engagement with her.

In an American study, Morse, *et al.* (2006) found that when the caregiver is not engaged with the sufferer this lack of engagement can be manifested as false pity, which can feel inappropriate to the patient and can cause anger. This took place in the interaction between Angie and Tamsin. Angie's perceived false pity was interpreted by Tamsin as a lack of empathy, and she felt increasingly angry as a result. As we become more experienced as nurses, we become more able to differentiate between the need for different levels of engagement and empathy. Not all individuals want to engage fully with someone they do not know very well, or they might feel embarrassed about their situation. At such times, knowing when to control the level of engagement and empathy, and when to be more factual or not so intense, can be less distressing to the patient.

An example of this could be when a school nurse deliberately minimises the amount of eye contact with an adolescent young girl who is expressing suicidal feelings. She might purposely carry on with nursing tasks and ask factual questions in order to help the young person to feel less in the spotlight and under pressure. This might encourage her to talk more and express more of her feelings than she would have done in a more traditional discussion on such serious issues. Young people often choose to divulge their true inner feelings with their parents or others when eye contact is compromised, for example when their mother is driving or busy with another task. They might also use texts and e-mails when a subject becomes uncomfortable for them. It is important for nurses to take the lead from the client or patient in terms of what level of engagement is wanted, and become more skilled at discussing emotional matters in a factual manner, or not face to face. This can increase the amount of information given and can reduce the level of discomfort or distress on the part of the patient or client.

We all think that we know ourselves, but do we see ourselves as others see us, or as we would like to be seen? Luft and Ingham (1955) (cited in Luft 1969) in their seminal work, developed a model of self-awareness to help identify four different aspects of knowledge of ourselves (*see* Table 2.1). We have developed this concept in Table 2.2 through an example of how the Johari window could be used in practice.

TABLE 2.1 Johari window

Open and visible Known to self and known to others	Blind and unknown to self Known only to others
Hidden to others but known to self Known only to self	Unknown to both self and others Known neither to self or others

Source: Luft and Ingham (1955)

TABLE 2.2 Example of the Johari window in practice

Open and visible	Blind and unknown to self
Known to self and known to others	Known only to others
Joan knows that she finds patients who misuse alcohol hard to care for. She thinks it is waste of healthcare resources when someone has made an active choice to misuse alcohol. Joan's colleague, Anne, knows this too because Joan has said this in relation to other patients	*Anne might also suspect that Joan sees drinking as a sign of weakness and that someone could easily change their drinking habits. Joan is not aware that she sees drinking as a sign of weakness*
Hidden to others but known to self	Unknown to both self and others
Known only to self	Known neither to self or others
Joan might know that she feels strongly about people who misuse alcohol because she grew up with a father who drank as a way of coping with life. He was not the strong father figure that she would have wanted	*Neither Joan, Anne, nor anyone else know that Joan has no respect for those who misuse alcohol*

The Johari window can be a helpful tool in increasing our level of self-awareness so that we can reduce the areas that are unknown to us. This can help us to know ourselves better, and allow us to enhance our ability to deliver empathetic care.

THOUGHTS FOR YOUR PRACTICE

- Have you ever let your own personal or professional thoughts or feelings affect how you speak to someone, or how you interact with them?
- Are there any situations that you feel would be a particular challenge to interacting with someone, or providing care for a patient/client?
- Can you think of any ways that you could anticipate such a situation?
- Can you think of any ways that you can improve your current practice in line with this?
- Are there any situations where you struggle to identify with those in your care?
- Can you think of any ways to start to resolve this?
- Are there any situations in which you find that full engagement with the patient is compromised?

- Have you any thoughts about how to enhance the engagement in these situations?
- Can you think of any situations when you purposely reduce the level of perceived engagement, in order to reduce patient distress?
- Can you think of any other situations when this could be appropriate?

How can we become more emotionally intelligent and can we become emotionally brilliant?

CASE STUDY 2.3

Raj was halfway through a busy shift in the trauma centre. It had been difficult to ensure that patients were being prioritised in a way that provided safe care for all those in the centre at that time. He went to the next cubicle and saw a frightened young girl looking up at him. He smiled reassuringly, and then looked at the admissions information. He saw that her name was Patience and that she had been brought to the centre by her friend, having taken a small overdose of aspirin. She had already vomited so he knew that there was no immediate cause for concern about her physical health. He knew that some of his colleagues were deeply resentful of the time 'wasted' with people who had knowingly harmed themselves. They felt that these were often not serious attempts, but 'cries for help' or attention. Raj himself felt that cries for help were just that, and that no one who was happy would want to do such a thing. He was, therefore, always careful to try to determine the reason for their emotional distress, as he was aware that it might be the only occasion that someone was able to seek that help. He was also aware of the high suicide and parasuicide rates in young people, and did not feel that patients who presented at the centre should be treated with anything other than sensitive care, regardless of how busy they were at the time.

Patience was only 14 years old, and yet she had felt the need to express her unhappiness in this way, and maybe she really did want to escape from her situation through death. He sat down next to her and touched her hand. She carried on looking at him with fear in her eyes. Then he saw that she was crying with no sound; she looked as if she had lost all hope. He started talking to her calmly; firstly by introducing himself and commenting on the fact that trauma centres were frightening places to be. Secondly, he then asked her what had made her feel so desperate and said that he was here to try to understand what was making life so bleak for her at the moment. He said that there was no need for anyone in her family to know what she told him, but that he might need to consult with colleagues, to try to get her the help she needed. She seemed to relax at this point and started to tell him that a male friend of her parents had forced himself on her sexually the previous night. He had told Patience that nobody would believe her if she told them about this – it would only make others feel negatively towards her.

Raj felt anger rising within him as he listened to Patience's story of what had been happening to her. He found that he was consciously having to keep calm and suppress his own feelings of disgust and anger against the man who had made her feel like this. He said that he could understand why she was so frightened and why she had taken the action that she had, but there were people who could help her. He asked how close she was to her parents and she said that they were very close and that they were outside now, worried about her. Together they worked out how she wanted to tell them about her ordeal, with him beside her, and she agreed to see someone who she could talk to about her feelings after she had been discharged. Just before he left to get her parents, she smiled for the first time and said, 'Thank you for taking the time to listen to me, and for taking me seriously and for being so understanding.'

Discussion

Once we have increased our level of self-awareness, which is a continuous process, we are in a position to use our communication skills to best effect. It is essential that nurses realise that communication is inevitable, irreversible and is a genuine skill (Sines, Appleby and Raymond 2001). Whatever a nurse does, whether they speak or not, they need to be aware that they are communicating in some way. Marion, in Case study 2.1, was communicating by her lack of communication with Judy at the start of their time together. Marion was seeing this as merely focusing on the task in hand, namely the computer, and was not meaning to be unwelcoming or dismissive towards Judy, but that is exactly how her communication came across. We need to use all our skills as communicators, at all times, to ensure that people feel valued. Different aspects of this communication process will be discussed throughout the book.

Empathy and identification with the person involved, coupled with self-awareness, are essential for effective communication. As nurses, we need to be genuine in our interest in the people in our care and regard them positively, whatever their needs, circumstances and lifestyle choices (Wondrak 1998). For example, different skills are needed in communicating with:

➤ individuals with mental health needs;
➤ people with particular conditions;
➤ older people;
➤ people of different genders;
➤ children;
➤ people of different cultures;
➤ people in traumatic situations.

It is essential for all nurses to realise that whatever they say or imply by the way that they communicate is irreversible. Patients, clients and their friends and relations will remember key situations, including what was said and done at that point, for the rest of their lives. In addition, previous experiences might colour their feelings about any care that they might need in the future. They might not want to access healthcare services due to a lack of confidence in the care that might be provided. They also might be frightened and stressed when they do have to access care. Alternatively, they could approach future healthcare situations with confidence, rather than apprehension, safe in the knowledge that in their previous experience they had felt valued, cared for and respected, and that there was genuine warmth. This is a heavy responsibility, so all nurses must appreciate the importance of communication in everything they say and do in their practice.

Raj was using all his advanced communication skills in this interaction with Patience. He knew that this might be his only opportunity to help her and, despite being busy, he knew it was important to prioritise time with her. He could identify with Patience's distress and then was able to demonstrate to her that he was fully engaged with her by the questions he asked, his use of therapeutic touch and his active listening skills. Through his non-judgemental attitude Raj was genuine in his interest in her and demonstrated that he respected and valued her as a person.

These are important components of emotional intelligence, which he also demonstrated through his recognition of Patience's feelings, as well as his own. Although he felt anger and distress on her behalf, he was able to control these emotions in a way that demonstrated his ability to cope with the stressors and pressures of his role and working environment. He therefore demonstrated emotional self-awareness. He was able to be assertive and understanding, and was able to act autonomously to help Patience feel confident in expressing her feelings and distress about what had happened to her. He took a problem-solving approach by trying to find out what she wanted to do, and then helped her to see a way forward to make this happen. He recognised that she really wanted to tell her parents about her ordeal, but was not sure that she could do this on her own. With his support she felt that she could make decisions and therefore felt much more positive as a result. This was a highly distressing situation, and Raj used all his emotional intelligence to find a way of helping her to feel confident that there were ways in which she could start on the long road to recovery.

Goleman (1996) sees emotional intelligence in terms of five domains:

1 Knowing one's emotions – self-awareness: recognising a feeling 'as it happens' is the keystone of emotional intelligence.
2 Managing emotions – handling feelings so they are appropriate is an ability that build on self-awareness.
3 Motivating oneself – marshalling emotions in the service of a goal is essential for paying attention, for self-motivation and mastery and for creativity.
4 Recognising emotions in others – empathy, another ability that builds on emotional self-awareness is the fundamental 'people skill'.
5 Handling relationships – the art of relationships is skill in managing emotions in others.

Applying Goleman's domains to Raj's emotional intelligence, we see that Raj:
➤ was emotionally self-aware;
➤ could change the way he interacted with Patience as it happened;
➤ managed his own feelings of anger as well as Patience's feelings of distress and fear;
➤ used these to maximum effect in bringing about as positive an outcome as was possible within the timeframe of the consultation;
➤ was empathetic and understanding.

Sparrow and Knight (2006) say that 'emotional intelligence integrates feeling, thinking and doing. It is the habitual practice of thinking about feeling and feeling about thinking when choosing what to do' (p. 29). They take this further by saying that 'although we all have the capacity to behave with emotional intelligence, most of the time most of us do not, because we have interferences (beliefs, attitudes and habits) which impede us from doing so' (p. 30). If Raj had allowed his colleagues' beliefs, attitudes and habits to impact on his professional practice, he would have dismissed Patience's attendance at the trauma centre as an attention seeking cry for help. He would not have been able to use his emotional intelligence to draw out the reasons for her overdose and would have missed a valuable opportunity to help her. It needs to be part of our habitual practice to 'think about what we are feeling' and 'feel about what we are thinking' in order to make emotionally intelligent decisions.

Sparrow and Knight (2006) go on to say that 'to act with emotional intelligence, we need to:

➤ notice feelings;
➤ pay attention to them;
➤ give them significance;
➤ think about them;
➤ take them into account in choosing what to do.

This applies to our own feelings and those of others' (p. 31).

Raj did respond to his feelings and realised that Patience was genuinely distressed and he let that lead him into prioritising time with her during a busy period in the trauma centre. He was therefore acting with emotional intelligence and, if we see emotional intelligence being on a continuum towards emotional brilliance, we can see that is exactly what he was demonstrating. Goleman (1996) says that the ultimate test of mastery of emotional brilliance is dealing with someone at the peak of rage. Strategies at that point could be distraction, empathy with their feelings and perspective, and drawing them into an alternative way of thinking that is more positive.

Raj was also demonstrating emotional brilliance because it is not easy to extract information from a reluctant young person at the best of times, and Patience was very distressed, embarrassed and traumatised. The emotional brilliance, which combined self-awareness and empathy concerning extremes of emotions that were directed towards a positive outcome, was a clear indication of Raj's excellence as a compassionate practitioner.

THOUGHTS FOR YOUR PRACTICE

- Have you ever said anything, or not said something, that you have regretted later?
- How did you come to terms with this?
- Has your practice changed as a result?
- If not, can you think of any ways in which it should?
- Think about your level of emotional intelligence; is there any part of your practice that would benefit from an enhanced level of emotional thinking?

- Can you think of a time when you used your skills of emotional intelligence to practise in a way that demonstrated emotional brilliance?
- If so, did you share this with others?
- If not, would you consider doing so now?

KEY THEME TWO – SENSITIVITY

CASE STUDY 2.4

Real life patient experience

I have suffered a number of miscarriages during the last eight years and have visited the same hospital on some occasions. On each of these visits I have been quite shocked at the lack of sensitivity shown by the members of staff who dealt with me. During my last visit in February of last year I was told that each time I went to the toilet I had to use a bed pan so that any 'product' could be collected. During the course of the afternoon I visited the toilet on three occasions as did another patient and at no time were the bed pans collected. When I mentioned it to a member of staff I was given to understand that I was making a fuss about something that could not be dealt with by very busy staff.

On being discharged I had to complete a form that required the 'mother's signature'. Having just experienced my fifth miscarriage and having never gone full term I found this quite upsetting at the time. I did speak to a registrar about these two matters and she was very sympathetic and assured me that she would mention my first problem at the next departmental meeting. However, she was unable to reassure me regarding the second matter since it had been discussed at a previous meeting and she felt that there was very little chance of the pro forma being changed to cater for patients such as myself (Web Site on Patient Opinion, ID 2471).

Discussion

A definition of sensitivity is 'awareness of the needs and emotions of others' (Merriam-Webster 2008). There is a moral dimension to sensitivity which Jordan (2007) discusses, seeing moral sensitivity as including 'dimensions such as interpreting others' reactions and feelings, having empathy and role-taking ability, understanding how one's actions can affect the welfare and expectations of both oneself and others, and making inferences from others' behaviour and responding appropriately to their reactions' (p. 326).

In this distressing situation it can be clearly seen that the patient was treated without any moral sensitivity at all, a point that she clearly makes. At no time was she given the opportunity to express her emotions or discuss what was important to her at this traumatic time. Her precious baby was referred to merely as a 'product' to be collected. The distress of losing her baby was compounded by the fact that the baby was not seen as a potential human life. She had the added trauma of being reminded visually of her loss each time she visited the toilet as the bedpans were not taken away between visits. Staff busyness was seen as an adequate excuse for this lack of sensitivity.

Furthermore, she had to sign a form as 'a mother' when she had never experienced motherhood, having had five miscarriages. This again was the height of insensitivity. Although the doctor she spoke to was sympathetic about both situations and could see the inappropriateness of these aspects of her experience, she felt powerless to initiate change to bring about increased sensitivity for future patients in similar situations. Systems that are supposed to support good care can be inflexible and there is a potential lack of scope to bring about change. As nurses we need to challenge insensitive care, whenever we see it. We should feel empowered to discuss issues directly with the individual practitioners concerned and to raise matters at higher levels within the organisational hierarchy to bring about strategic change, as needed.

It is important to remember that once an individual needs care they become a patient and their individuality can be severely compromised. They become dependent on others, who they may have never have met before, for all their fundamental needs. This patient, who was normally fit and well, became dependent on others due to her miscarriage and there was no evidence of the compassionate, sensitive care that she should have received. This resulted in her not being seen as an individual who was bereaved and traumatised, but as someone who was 'making a fuss'. People have a right to expect that their vulnerability at times of illness will be understood, whether this is temporary and short-lived or more severe and long-standing. We all feel vulnerable, isolated and powerless in unknown situations where we feel out of control. We could easily feel that we are 'a problem' and become reluctant to express our needs, and therefore be at danger of losing our personal identity. This would be particularly true should we be faced with nurses who are indifferent, and who lack empathy, caring, sensitivity and warmth. In addition, as nurses we need to ensure that we retain our humility and kindness, as well as our empathy, as discussed earlier in the chapter.

Sensitivity, in terms of nursing practice, also involves ensuring that people feel comfortable in the care setting and therefore the concept of 'emotional comfort' is key to this. We will now discuss this as a central focus in relation to sensitive care, along with the importance of recognising the 'professional artistry' of nursing, if we practise with true compassion. Using humour in a sensitive, therapeutic manner within nursing care will then be discussed. Finally we will discuss whether sensitive nursing care is possible within the financial climate that affects so much of healthcare today. We need to find ways of retaining sensitive and compassionate care, despite the very real financial pressures that are often such strong drivers in how we deliver our nursing care.

Do we understand the importance of emotional comfort and the appropriate use of humour?

CASE STUDY 2.5

Ling could see that Winston was not as relaxed and full of jokes as he normally was. He appeared to be worried and she could see that he was trying to find a way to discuss something with her. Ling had been visiting Winston and his wife, Stella, for some months now and she felt that she had got to know them quite well. Her many previous years working in hospitals, then the community, had taught her a great deal about how different people express their anxiety, and she could see that Winston was uneasy today. Stella had been becoming increasingly dependent on carers over the previous months, including Winston, and it was clear that her health was deteriorating. Winston and Stella had always been emotionally very close and she knew how worried he was about losing her. They were quite mutually dependent on each other, emotionally and physically, and she was worried how he would cope as Stella's situation deteriorated.

Ling sat down to indicate that she was not in a hurry, despite the fact that she had many more visits to do that morning. Sometimes there was only one opportunity for a sensitive discussion, as this was likely to be, and it was important to seize that opportunity. She started by saying that he looked worried and obviously had something on his mind and asked whether there was anything he wanted to talk about. He said that he was aware that Stella was becoming less and less able to move easily and that the carer had indicated earlier in the day that there might be more disruption at night as Stella's needs increased. Therefore he might want to consider sleeping in separate beds. He really did not want to be parted from her at night. With tears in his eyes, he said that he knew that he would soon lose her and he wanted to make the most of every minute that they had left together.

He said, 'Just because there might be more comings and goings at night that's no reason for us to be apart. We've been through worse in our lives, and love and marriage are for better, for worse, in sickness and in health. I can cope with that if she can cope with all that she has to.' He then smiled and said, 'I would miss her if she wasn't there every night, although she does snore and has cold feet and tries to take all the sheets and blankets in the middle of the night. If you could make it so that she can stay in our bed, and sort out her grabbing the covers in the night, that would make me feel a lot better.'

Ling recognised the seriousness of the message Winston was giving, despite his attempt at humour. She knew that separation every night would be detrimental to them both. She knew the value and importance of the marital bed as a time for physical and emotional intimacy and could sense that Winston saw this as the start of their gradual separation and he did not want that, and was not ready to let her go – even just at night. Ling said, 'Well let's make a deal. I will think about ways to reduce the problems in relation to her increasing needs and you sort out her taking all the bed clothes at night.'

Ling promised to come back to discuss Stella's future needs, and how that would impact on their lives, and Winston's role in this. He looked relieved, and as a man who found it difficult to express his feelings, she knew that expressing these thoughts had been hard for him. He usually found ways of expressing things with humour, as he had done today, and it was important that she responded in the same way. They both understood each other well enough to know that an important worry had been raised and responded to today. She was very glad that she had prioritised this discussion within her busy day. She saw the smile come back to his face, and the way that he joked with her when she left reassured her that he was feeling much more positive than at the start of her visit.

Discussion

Ling was highly experienced and knew Winston and his situation well, so she was able to sense his unease or emotional discomfort. In an Australian study, Williams and Irurita (2004) describe emotional discomfort as unpleasant or negative feelings or a state of tension. Winston was tense and uneasy and Ling clearly understood this and sensed his feelings of negativity about Stella's deteriorating situation. It was important for Ling to try to minimise Winston's feelings of discomfort, and also to try to make him feel emotionally comfortable.

Williams and Irurita (2004) say that 'emotional comfort' minimises physical discomfort and involves patient participation in recovery. They say that the patient's perception of personal control is a central feature of emotional comfort (Williams and Irurita 2006). Winston was starting to feel that he was no longer in control of his and Stella's destiny and was very unsettled by this. By the time Ling left, Winston had moved from a state of emotional discomfort to that of emotional comfort, which Williams and Irurita (2004) describe as 'pleasant, positive feelings; a state of relaxation that affects the physical status of the body' (p. 809).

They say that the mind and the body are inextricably linked, therefore emotional stress will increase physical manifestations of illness and these same physical symptoms could cause emotional distress. Winston would not want his level of anxiety to affect Stella, either physically or emotionally.

Ling was able to help Winston make that transition to emotional comfort by increasing his **level of security** because she was a competent, experienced practitioner, who had a strong relationship with the couple. She was also intending to increase his **level of knowing** through giving him more information and discussing what to expect and what to do as Stella's situation evolved. Ling also increased Winston's **level of personal value** by recognising his personal identity and the fact that there was a disruption of personal choice and control over both their normal activities and routines. These levels are highlighted by Williams and Irurita (2004) as important components of promoting emotional comfort. Providing emotional comfort is an important part of the art of nursing.

Nursing can be seen as an integration of art and science. Ling was clearly using her skills in relation to the art of nursing. Carper (1978), in her seminal text, perceives nursing as both an art and a science, and said that there was an increasing emphasis on the empirical or scientific aspects of nursing. The emphasis on highly technological nursing care has increased exponentially since this time. Nurses have increased the evidence base of their practice and their knowledge and technological skills, which are in the realms of the science of nursing. Potentially this could be perceived to be to the detriment of their nursing skills within the art of nursing (Carper 1978). The art of nursing takes into account empathy and sensitivity, self-awareness, intuition and the therapeutic use of self.

Intuition can be seen as the advanced form of reasoning of an expert practitioner and involves working in partnership with patients. Ling was clearly demonstrating her intuition in knowing that it was important to Winston to talk to her that day. She was also aware of his emotional discomfort and the need to work with him to find solutions for his concerns. Benner (1984) and Benner and Tanner (1987) discuss the importance of intuition as part of expert practice. Ling was practising as an expert nurse, using all her empathy, sensitivity and therapeutic use of self. She also saw the uniqueness of Winston, his relationship with Stella and their overall situation. Ling was therefore using professional artistry within her interaction with Winston.

Schon (1987) defines professional artistry as 'the competence by which practitioners handle indeterminate zones of practice; however that competence may relate to technical rationality' (p. 13). So he clearly recognises the need for scientific, or evidence-based, practice, but also focuses on the professional artistry in responding sensitively and appropriately to individual patients' needs, and responding flexibly to their changing circumstances. Ling, during this visit, was focusing more on the fact finding, using the artistic and empathetic aspects of nursing. When she returns to Winston and Stella she might focus more on the problem solving, and potentially more scientific components of Stella's care. These should be inextricably linked in any interaction with patients.

The art of nursing is less measurable and less clearly articulated than the more scientific aspects of nursing. However, Lumby (cited in Rose and Parker 1994) says:

> I see this art every time I walk into an environment where a nurse is busy 'creating' the day for another person. They are busy using light, space, sound, words, movement and touch to deliver the message of care . . . perhaps nursing as an art can only be recognised if the ward is viewed as a concert hall and the patients the audience. (p. 1009)

In the case study, Ling was using words and humour as the instruments in her art, and it would be possible for anyone observing her interaction with Winston to see that she was using her professional artistry to good effect.

Ling also used gentle humour in her interaction with Winston. This was initiated by him and she took the lead from him. Ling is an experienced nurse, and had a good relationship with Winston, so knew how to use humour appropriately in this situation. It is sometimes appropriate to use humour in nursing care, but it needs to be used carefully, in order to improve rapport and not to make people feel undervalued. It is possible for nurses to use humour in a mocking way, that makes people feel stupid and that feelings are abnormal or that their expectations for the future are unrealistic. For example, a nurse could use humour in a very negative way to mock someone with a learning disability wanting to have a relationship with someone of the opposite gender.

When humour is used appropriately, patients can find this therapeutic and the whole experience of care more enjoyable, as the following patient experiences show.

> The consultants at the hospitals have been kind, sympathetic and extremely professional at all times, enabling me to be at ease whether happy, sad, confused or lost. Above all, every member of staff has been courteous, kind and had a smashing sense of humour (is it on the job description?). (Web Site on Patient Opinion, ID 7904)

> All of the staff (nursing staff and theatre staff) worked together quickly, smoothly and without fuss. My operation was carried out on time and successfully. This treatment continued throughout my stay on the ward. I was treated with dignity, politeness, humour (where appropriate) and care and the whole visit was much more pleasant than I had anticipated. Everyone I came in contact with made me feel that I was important to them, not just a number. I even enjoyed the food! (Web Site on Patient Opinion, ID 3661)

In a study in Ireland, McCabe (2004) linked friendliness and the use of humour, and found that nurses who use humour are perceived by patients to be more approachable. They found that the use of humour raised patients' self-esteem and the use of humour on a children's ward could have the effect of reducing stress. The release of endorphins through laughter could reduce stress in staff, patients and carers. A study undertaken at Indiana State University and the University of South Florida (Bennett and Lengacher 2008) found that smiles and laughter help the body to produce antibodies to protect against infection and reduce pain, and could speed up recovery times. In addition, it increases the level of endorphins, the body's natural painkillers, and can lower levels of the stress hormone cortisol. Tension, anger and worry make people more vulnerable to infections; whereas laughter can reduce symptoms of allergies and the pain of arthritis sufferers, and can also lower blood pressure.

However, two studies in Finland and America (Astedt-Kurki and Isola 2001; Sumners 1990) have highlighted that changes in practice have reduced the amount of contact with patients. Nurses can be in a good position to have sustained contact with patients. This sustained contact builds relationships in which humour can be used therapeutically. However, if contact with patients is reduced, nurses do not have the time to build such relationships and this can mean that humour is not used at all, or is used inappropriately. Therefore the opportunity to use humour therapeutically is greatly compromised. An opportunity to reduce anxiety, pain and muscular tension and enhance physical and psychological well-being through the use of humour can be lost. The patients in these studies also felt that humour made nurses more approachable and it helped to build up a rapport between them and the nursing staff. As a result, patients felt that togetherness, warmth, friendliness and closeness developed.

From the nurses' perspective, they saw the use of humour as a form of communication. This helped them cope with difficult situations and enhanced their problem solving and creativity. Humour also helped to reduce conflict and intensify their interactions with patients. However, it is important to recognise that humour is only perceived as therapeutic if it is interpreted that way by the patient or client.

Nurses use 'black humour', or an in-house common language, to help them cope with illness and the loss of patients. Therefore, this can be seen as not necessarily demonstrating a lack of compassion, but as a way of maintaining humanity and compassion within nursing practice. Astedt-Kurki and Isola (2001) and Sumners (1990) also found that more mature or experienced nurses were more able to use humour in their nursing care. However, it is important to remember that 'humour is unique to each person and culture. What one individual may feel humorous may shock another' (Astedt-Kurki and Isola 2001, p. 453). They also say that 'humour must never violate the patient's human dignity' (p. 458). Sumners (1990) stresses the importance of humour being used appropriately and says that it 'needs to be used judiciously and with knowledge' (p. 200).

THOUGHTS FOR YOUR PRACTICE

- Have you ever felt vulnerable as a patient and at risk of losing your identity?
- Did you feel that your usual ability to be assertive deserted you in this situation?
- What made you feel this way?
- Can you identify patients who could have felt very vulnerable in your care setting?
- Could you do anything to help them feel less vulnerable?
- How could you ensure that your nursing care increases your patients' emotional comfort?
- Think of some times when you have used your intuition to respond more effectively to situations with patients.
- Try to think of ways where you could use your intuition to greater effect.
- Think of a situation when you focused more on the science of nursing.
- Think of a situation when you focused more on the art of nursing.
- Do you feel that there ways that you could use both the art and science of nursing in a more integrated way in your practice?
- Can you think of times when humour helped you to build rapport and strengthened your relationships with patients?
- Can you think of times when humour would have been inappropriate?
- Can you think of times when you saw humour being used inappropriately?
- Can you think of a time when humour was used therapeutically?
- Do you think that you could use therapeutic humour more in your day-to-day practice?

Sensitive care and resources – is there a conflict?

CASE STUDY 2.6

Real life patient experience

Sitting for long periods by a mute patient, as I did, meant that I looked around at the ebb and flow of staff activity. Although the open corner nursing station means that staff can no longer withdraw into a closed office, this new arrangement gives an illusion of engagement with, and efficient observation of, nearby patients (who are only a few yards away). I watched carefully what was happening minute by minute.

Staff milled around the station. Some interacted with one another. Some were doing paper work. Some were permanently transfixed by a computer screen. Any contact with any patient (which was sparse compared to this station-centred, staff-centred activity) emerged in the main because a relative requested it (leaving me wondering what happens when relatives are absent).

One old gentleman, who was sitting up and speaking, but not ambulant, asked the nurse for a bottle, and who, in our presence, said, 'Sorry love – haven't got time.' He became so upset that my wife (another ex-nurse) went to get him one and pulled his screens around.

It is as if there is an invisible wall, about a yard from the nursing station, which closes the awareness of the staff into a sort of bubble. This seemed to me to be like what we now know of the dangers of mobile phones in public spaces, where drivers and foot passengers put all at risk because their attention is in a tunnel and oblivious to the immediate environment.

The above lists suggest that care on this ward is simply not good enough. If it were only on this ward then it would be serious, but at least rectifiable in the future (by corrective staff training and regular audits). My worry is that it reflects a more general change in the ethos of nursing.

Trained nurses now seem to be obsessed by recording activity than the activity itself. Humane direct tending of patients seems to have been devolved to care assistants. That leaves it to chance about the sensitivity, common sense and common decency of these individuals one by one. This matter of the care of dying people should not be left to chance – nursing supposedly has, over time, elevated the care process to an art ('the nursing process', 'holistic care', 'patient-centred care').

Despite these claims, what we witnessed was the antithesis of these aspirations, so that they now look like empty rhetorical claims. What we witnessed overall was the opposite of patient-centred care. The only crumb of comfort was that in the odd honest conversation, some of the trained staff admitted that their profession has lost its way about standards of care. Maybe then, a starting point is that this hospital and others in the NHS need an honest appraisal of what nursing standards are for severely disabled and dying patients.

> A good question to pose to all staff, from the CEO and Director of Nursing downwards, is this: 'Would I want to be cared for on this ward?' (Web Site on Patient Opinion, ID 7826)

Discussion

This distressing situation, which has been recorded exactly as it was written on the Patient Opinion web site, is written from the point of view of a visitor, and is traumatic to read. He is obviously referring to knowledge gained from his wife's experience as an ex-nurse, and it is unclear but he could be an ex-nurse himself. He is clearly appalled at the care he has witnessed and raises many important issues about sensitivity of care in relation to available resources.

The nursing station, although positioned for maximum observation of patients, appears to be isolated behind an 'invisible wall'. He differentiates between activities that are staff-centred and nursing station-centred, and those that are patient-centred. He says that a lot of what he sees is staff-centred and administration-orientated and that nurses seem to resent interruptions. They appear not to have time to meet the fundamental needs of the vulnerable people in their care, and they seem to focus more on recording activities, rather than the care itself. He implies that there is insufficient training and supervision of the care assistants, who appear to be delivering most of this care. He questions standards of nursing care and asks whether the people in charge of the hospital would want to be cared for on this ward.

Although there are different explanations for this situation and different perspectives involved, the message is clear that patients are not being cared for in a sensitive manner, and that too much emphasis is being placed on administrative tasks, to the detriment of hands-on care.

In an English study, Foster and Hawkins (2005) say that the increase in technology can give nurses reasons to stay away from the patient's bedside, or make care task-orientated, with no communication established with the patient. They say that nurses can 'spend more time monitoring the collection of data than engaging with the physical and emotional care of the patient' (p. 700). This appears to be the case in the situation described, and, in fact, Ford (2008) suggests that some nurses say that there is such an emphasis on bed management, cost effectiveness, funding and meeting targets that there are just not the resources to meet fundamental care needs.

However, Foster and Hawkins (2005) also say that this increase in technology could potentially be a really positive development, because it could increase the amount of time available for direct nursing care, due to there being less task-orientated activities that need to take place. This time could be used to build relationships with patients and enhance emotional well-being and comfort, through the use of therapeutic touch and empathetic relationships that encourage people to self-disclose.

Some of the points raised in this section highlight either thoughtless, or perhaps even intentional, insensitive care. However, there are times when the most sensitive of nurses feel that they are unable to provide the quality of care that they believe is right. They become deeply distressed by their perceived failure to meet the patient's or client's needs. This moral distress is described in a joint Ugandan and Canadian study by Fournier, *et al.* (2007) who say that there are many challenges to nurses providing effective or compassionate care, which cause 'moral distress'(p. 262). This can cause nurses to leave their posts and to suffer from 'burn out' (p. 263). Resource constraints can make compassionate care prohibitive. Other challenges to sensitive care can be poverty, fear of contagion and lack of ongoing education, which are factors in the delivery of care in developing countries, such as Uganda. Nurses feel disempowered and lack control over exacerbating factors in relation to health, and are unable to provide the care they feel the patient deserves and needs.

A Norwegian study by Hem and Heggen (2004) uses the parable of the Good Samaritan to demonstrate that nurses have a moral responsibility to care for the sick and their illness can be compounded by the individual's helplessness, vulnerability and suffering. In the parable, the Good Samaritan feels pity for the plight of the suffering man and goes to his aid, rather than passing by on the other side of the road. Using this example, it is clear that nurses do have a moral responsibility for patients in their care, and they can feel real distress when patients' need for care is not met. Desensitisation can be used as a means of coping with the uncopeable, and nurses can lose their empathy and sensitivity, and therefore their compassion, within their nursing practice.

Patients used to spend more time in hospital and there was more time to build up relationships. Building a therapeutic relationship is a complex process that takes time, both at any given point and over a period of time. Therefore nurses need to seize every opportunity to develop therapeutic, patient-centred relationships that lie at the heart of sensitive, compassionate care.

A patient-centred approach does not necessarily mean that nurses need to spend hours with patients; it is more about the quality of the time spent together. For example, a nurse who is changing an intravenous infusion bag can change the bag in a task-orientated manner that includes little or no com-munication with the patient. Alternatively she can smile, put a hand on the patient's shoulder and take time to talk with the patient, assess for altered health status and provide reassurance. Nurses have been criticised for talking about their social lives while carrying out nursing care, and it is clear that if they are finding time to discuss personal issues, they could use this time to better effect to discuss issues important to the patient.

THOUGHTS FOR YOUR PRACTICE

- Have you seen insensitive care in your area of practice?
- On reflection, do you feel that you have ever been more insensitive to your patients' needs and emotions than you would ever intend to be?
- Do you feel that you can challenge insensitive care in your practice area?
- Do you feel able to influence processes and resourcing on a strategic level?
- Could you do more to ensure that your patients receive sensitive care?
- Do you ever feel that it is difficult to deliver sensitive care within your practice?
- If so, what are the reasons for this?
- Do you ever feel distressed about the fact that you cannot always deliver the sensitive care you would like to?
- How do you deal with these emotions?

SUMMARY – LINKS TO COMPASSION AND CARING

We hope that we have raised issues within this chapter that have challenged your understanding of concepts in relation to empathy and sensitivity. We believe that self-awareness is the starting point to understanding what it means to engage with people in an empathetic manner within your nursing role. If we do not know ourselves, then how can we understand the needs of others? Nurses need to become not only emotional intelligent, but also emotionally brilliant practitioners. Even if we are skilled and emotionally brilliant nurses, this can be compromised in certain situations by our own norms and values, and by those of others. We need to work towards minimising the chances of this happening, and maximising our potential for providing emotionally brilliant empathetic and compassionate care.

Sensitive care involves providing an environment for emotional comfort.

This involves practising in a way that combines the art and science of nursing and capitalises on our ability to use professional artistry within our interaction with people. Humour can be used therapeutically by skilled and experienced practitioners, and this can aid recovery and reduce the manifestations of illness, as long as it is used with care. Technological advances and financial constraints have the potential to lead us into a more task-orientated approach to nursing care. However, external forces and financial constraints can only be blamed for insensitive care up to a point. We are all accountable and responsible for our actions and omissions in terms of the nursing care we provide.

Patients, clients and residents need to be confident that they will be treated with empathy and sensitivity, and in ways that do not compromise their dignity and privacy. Some things cost nothing; for example, it takes no time to greet someone with a smile and their preferred name and to ensure that each interaction is as patient-orientated as possible.

REFERENCES

Astedt-Kurki P, Isola A. Humour between nurse and patient, and among staff: analysis of nurses' diaries. *J Adv Nurs*. 2001; **35**(3): 452–8.

Benner P. *From Novice to Expert: excellence and power in clinical nursing practice*. Menlo Park, CA: Addison-Wesley Publishing Company; 1984.

Benner P, Tanner C. Clinical judgement: how expert nurses use intuition. *Am J Nurs*. 1987; **87**(1): 23–31.

Bennett M, Lengacher C. Humor and laughter may influence health: III. Laughter and health outcomes. *Evid Based Complement Alternat Med*. 2008; **5**(1); 37–40.

Carper B. Fundamental patterns of knowing in nursing. *Adv Nurs Sci*. 1978; **1**(1): 13–23.

Ford P. Dignity: the heart of nursing. *RCN magazine*. 2008; Spring: 26–7.

Foster T, Hawkins J. The therapeutic relationship: dead or merely impeded by technology. *BJN*. 2005; **14**(13): 698–702.

Fournier B, Kipp W, Mill J, *et al*. The nursing care of AIDS patients in Uganda. *J Transcult Nurs*. 2007; **18**(3): 257–64.

Goleman D. *Emotional Intelligence*. London: Bloomsbury; 1996.

Hem M, Heggen K. Is compassion central to nursing practice? *Contemp Nurse*. 2004; **17**(1–2): 19–31.

Jordan J. Taking the first step toward a moral action: a review of moral sensitivity measurement across domains. *J Genet Psychol*. 2007; **168**(3): 323–9.

Kirschenbaum H, Henderson V. *The Carl Rogers Readers*. London: Constable; 1990.

Luft J, Ingham H (1955). The Johari window: a graphic model of interpersonal awareness. In: Luft J, editor. *Of Human Interaction*. Palo Alto: California National Press; 1969.

McCabe C. Nurse-patient communication: an exploration of patients' experiences. *J Clin Nurs*. 2004; **13**(1): 41–9.

McCabe C, Timmins F. *Communication Skills For Nursing Practice*. Basingstoke: Palgrave MacMillan; 2006.

Merriam-Webster. *Online Dictionary*. Available at: www.merriam-webster.com/dictionary/sensitivity (accessed 30 April 2008).

Moore L. Empathy: a clinician's perspective. *The ASHA Leader*. **11**(10): 16–17; 34–5.

Morse J, Bottorff J, Anderson G, *et al.* Beyond empathy: expanding expressions of caring. *J Adv Nurs*. 2006; **53**(1): 75–87.

Reynolds W, Scott P. Nursing, empathy and perception of the moral. *J Adv Nurs*. 2000; **32**(1): 235–42.

Rose P, Parker D. Nursing: an integration of art and science within the experience of the practitioner. *J Adv Nurs*. 1994; **20**(6): 1004–10.

Rungapadiachy D. *Interpersonal Communication and Psychology for Healthcare Professionals*. Oxford: Butterworth Heinemann; 1999.

Schon D. *Educating the Reflective Practitioner*. San Francisco, CA: Jossey-Bass; 1987.

Sines D, Appleby F, Raymond E. *Community Health Care Nursing*. Oxford: Blackwell Science; 2001.

Sparrow T, Knight A. *Applied EI: the importance of attitudes in developing emotional intelligence*. Chichester: John Wiley and Sons Ltd; 2006.

Sumners A. Professional nurses' attitudes towards humour. *J Adv Nurs*. 1990; **15**(2): 196–200.

Williams A, Irurita V. Therapeutic and non-therapeutic interpersonal interactions: the patient's perspective. *J Clin Nurs*. 2004; **13**(7): 806–15.

Williams A, Irurita V. Emotional comfort: the patient's perspective of a therapeutic context. *Int J Nurs Stud*. 2006; **43**(4): 405–15.

Wondrak R. *Interpersonal Skills for Nurses and Health Care Professionals*. Oxford: Blackwell Science; 1998.

www.britannica.com/eb/article-9032549/empathy

www.patientopinion.org.uk/opinion.aspx?opinionID=2471

www.patientopinion.org.uk/opinion.aspx?opinionID=3661

www.patientopinion.org.uk/opinion.aspx?opinionID=7826

www.patientopinion.org.uk/opinion.aspx?opinionID=7904

CHAPTER 3

Dignity and respect

Overview of the chapter

OVERVIEW OF THE CHAPTER

Having discussed the importance of empathy and sensitivity in nursing care, the next challenge is to recognise the importance of treating patients and clients with the dignity and respect they deserve. Patients and clients cannot receive compassionate care without a strong focus on these essential aspects of nursing. This chapter aims to help you understand what dignity is, and is not, as well as helping you to consider other aspects of respect within your interactions and practice.

It is sometimes easier to identify when dignity is not central to nursing practice, but we need to increase our understanding of what this actually means to patients and nurses. These perspectives can be very different and can be influenced by changing healthcare priorities. The building of trusting and therapeutic, patient-centred relationships, of which non-judgemental attitude is a key component, is essential in relation to patients and clients feeling that they are being treated with respect. It is essential that dignity and respect are put at the top of the nursing agenda.

KEY THEME ONE – DIGNITY

CASE STUDY 3.1

Marjorie had been admitted to hospital with a urinary tract infection. Normally she managed to care for herself at home, despite the relentless advancing multiple sclerosis that affected everything she did. She hated being in hospital and found that attitudes and care varied enormously from nurse to nurse and ward to ward.

She hated being dependent on others for help, but outside her home environment with unfamiliar circumstances and more distant toilet facilities, she had to accept that receiving help was inevitable.

She woke up one night with an increasing need to go to the toilet. She rang her bell reluctantly because she knew that the nurses hated to be disturbed at night. She waited for 10 minutes, which passed like an eternity, looking at her watch more and more frequently. She rang the bell again, afraid that she would wet the bed – something she had never done in her life. Eventually a male nurse appeared and she asked him for a commode. He sighed and asked, 'Is it for number one or number two?' She answered timidly that she just wanted to pass urine. He answered brusquely, 'Then do it in your pad as the commode is only for number two during the night.' He then walked quickly out of her bay.

Marjorie lay there for over an hour in increasing discomfort and pain, crying quietly, until she could not cope any longer and had to let go of her bladder. She was absolutely mortified as soon as she felt the relief from emptying her bladder. She lay there, awake until morning, thinking about what life had come to, that she was reduced to lying in her own urine all night. She had to get out of this place as quickly as possible and vowed not to accept being sent to hospital again, however bad her symptoms were. She did not want to feel this humiliated ever again and was so upset that she had been made to feel this way.

Discussion

It is clear from Case study 3.1 that Marjorie's dignity was severely compromised. She was in a highly dependent situation, which was traumatic enough for such a self-sufficient woman. However, the way she was made to feel over a normal human function, which was the reason she had been admitted in the first place, made her feel devalued. Passing urine is a private and personal activity and the nurse's attitude was dismissive and demeaning, and showed no understanding of her situation, her medical condition or Marjorie as an individual. This will have a lifelong effect on her desire to accept future care.

It can sometimes be easier to identify when dignity is not central to care or communication, than to truly identify what dignity actually means. Lewis (2006) says that 'undignified care is associated with invisibility, depersonalisation and treatment of the individual as an object' (p. 2). He also says that this can involve humiliation and abuse as well as narrow and mechanistic approaches to care. He continues: 'People can't necessarily define it but they know when it isn't there' (p. 2). Michael Parkinson, Dignity Ambassador for the Dignity in Care campaign in the UK, agrees that dignity is difficult to define. He suggests, 'Dignity is a strange word, with connotations of pomp and privilege. Maybe "compassion" is a better word' (Parkinson 2008, p. 14). A definition that could be helpful is, 'a state, quality, or manner worthy of esteem or respect, and self-respect' (Merriam-Webster 2008).

It can be clearly seen that Marjorie's care did involve humiliation and abuse of her rights as an individual. She had personal needs concerning normal human activities, and at that point she was unable to function independently. The nurse involved appeared more concerned with what was easier for him, and did not see Marjorie as a person in her own right. He certainly was not treating her with compassion or respect.

Parkinson (2008) emphasises the importance of older people in stabilising society through their experience and knowledge, and the importance of this intergenerational effect. He talks about the distress of seeing how his mother, in the latter stages of dementia, was not treated with dignity by her carers. She was neglected in terms of hygiene and she was exposed to experiences that she would have found distressing. She was nursed in a mixed sex ward alongside men who were similarly disorientated and who exposed themselves on a frequent basis. He says that she was not valued as an individual nor treated with humanity by many. He sees the ultimate in respect as nursing staff that did care and took the time to attend her funeral. He says that it is important to recognise older people's knowledge and life experiences and use this as an inspiration to younger people. He says that we should be ashamed of the current lack of dignity, respect and compassion in the care of older people in the United Kingdom. Some cultures appear to treat their elders with reverence and respect, but this is not always the case. Older people can feel that society treats them as useless and invisible, a drain on the economy and a problem in terms of providing care for them. Is this the way we want people who have contributed so much throughout their lives to be treated?

What does dignity mean to patients and clients?

CASE STUDY 3.2

Constantine was feeling particularly agitated this morning. She was coping with her withdrawal from heroin and crack as well as she could and in some ways it was not as hard as she had feared. She had not felt ready to embark on the traumatic and sudden stopping of the drugs that she saw as the only way to cope with the pressures of life, and had been really afraid to take this major step. However, when she was arrested after a police raid of her boyfriend's flat, which involved an overnight stay with the police, she thought that she would at least try to stop taking drugs.

She was now in a residential substance misuse centre. The staff there were being very supportive and she was starting to feel that she might be able to manage without drugs. However, although she understood the reasons for this, she hated the restrictions on her personal independence. She knew that she did not feel safe without these restrictions at the moment, and that rules had to be obeyed in order to keep herself and others safe and as likely to succeed as possible. She also knew that she needed to be tested frequently and randomly for signs of drugs in her system, and she did not resent this at all. What she did resent was the fact this involved testing her urine, and the passing of the sample had to be observed in order to be sure that it was genuinely hers. She knew more than most just how devious people with a drug habit could be, and that taking samples of others' urine into the toilet, so that this could be tested as their own, was very common practice. However, being watched on the toilet, often by a male nurse, was something she could not come to terms with.

Max, the male nurse who accompanied her to the toilet on this particular morning, was clearly highly uncomfortable with the process too. He was trying to give her privacy as much as was possible while still making sure that the specimen was actually hers. She told him how difficult she felt this was and how she felt that the whole process compromised her dignity and he agreed. She said that many others felt the same. He explained to her that it was possible to take saliva samples, which was less intrusive. However, these would not give immediate results as the lab they would be sent to could not send back results in much under a week. He also explained how expensive this would be.

Constantine felt that she had his support, though, when he said that he felt that her dignity and that of others was being compromised. He promised to take this forward to a management meeting and she felt confident that he would.

After she left the centre, she later found out, when she was supporting another user of the service who had recently stopped taking drugs, that the system had changed and saliva samples were now taken instead. She felt pleased to have been part of this change and was very pleased that Max had kept his word and managed to bring about this change based purely on the grounds of dignity, despite the financial pressures on the service.

Discussion

It is important to identify what patients actually perceive as dignity, or what we ourselves would view as dignified care. Reporting on a New Zealand study, Carter, *et al.* (2004) say that dignity from a patient's perspective is perceived in terms of the relationship between the maintenance of hope, increasing dependence and the need to ask for help. The study found that the manner in which people responded to these needs was fundamental to maintaining dignity.

It is clear that Marjorie in Case study 3.1 was not responded to in a way that promoted her dignity. However, in contrast, Constantine's situation in Case study 3.2 clearly demonstrates that nurses did respond to patients' concerns about a loss of dignity, and systems were changed as a result – even though this meant that the service had to bear additional financial costs and there had to be compromises in terms of the speed of results being available to staff.

Constantine and her fellow users of the mental health service were clear that compromising privacy was compromising their dignity and therefore this needed to be addressed. Nursing staff also took this view and took an active role in effecting a change in practice. Privacy, or the lack of it, is also discussed by Charles-Edwards and Brotchie (2005) in relation to the nursing of children. They identify three ways in which privacy can be perceived.

1 **Physical privacy**, which involves protecting modesty, avoiding embarrassment over bodily functions and respect when carrying out invasive procedures.
2 **Information privacy**, which includes confidentiality in relation to children and how this can compromise the rights of parents. Children and their parents have to be seen as separate identities, as their concerns and priorities might be different.
3 **Family privacy**, where the family has freedom of unwarranted interference by the State. This last point obviously has to be viewed with sensitivity and the child's well-being has to be treated as paramount. Children, traditionally, have not been seen as having their own privacy needs, and therefore their dignity, in terms of being respected in their own right, could have been compromised.

People who misuse drugs or alcohol, like Constantine, could easily be seen as people who are undeserving of respect and privacy, as could prisoners, women or men who work on the streets, or anyone else who has different priorities and lifestyles to us.

When visiting a day centre, Lewis (2006) found that older people had strong feelings about what dignity meant to them. They said that it meant being recognised as a person, being listened to and being understood when they said what was important to them. They wanted to be treated as if they were the only person in the world, with people taking time to get to know them. They wanted nurses to be flexible in allowing sufficient time and interaction to take place and for them to realise that, although they may be frail and vulnerable, they are not just someone to be 'cured' and moved on (p. 2).

Constantine, although not an older person, felt the same way. She wanted to be respected as a person and listened to in terms of what was important to her. Although Max's presence in the toilet was compulsory, he used the time to good effect by listening to her concerns, and treating her as an individual. More than this, although he knew that she would not be with the service for very much longer, he took her concerns seriously by moving the service forward to promote a greater focus on dignity.

In studies by Walsh and Kowanko (2002) and Shotton and Seedhouse (1998), patients said that they felt their care was not dignified; not only when they were inappropriately dressed or covered, but also when there was inadequate allocation of time or resources, or acknowledgement of their views and feelings.

A key time when people are deeply concerned about a potential loss of dignity is when they are nearing the end of their lives. Many people feel that they want to have some control over where and how they die, particularly if their health is deteriorating and death is inevitable. Assisted death is a very contentious subject, and one which attracts very strong views. If the patient is the central focus, their views need to be listened to and not influenced by the practitioners' beliefs and values. In Oregon, an Act was passed in 1997 called the Death with Dignity Act. The 2007 summary based on the Act (Oregon State Web site 2007) found that the most common end-of-life concerns were loss of autonomy (100%), decreasing ability to participate in activities that made life enjoyable (86%), loss of dignity (86%) and fears about inadequate pain control (33%). It would be interesting to compare the concerns these patients raised with those of patients across the world to see whether they are the same in other countries with different cultures. There are different cultural and religious views about assisted death. Many religions are not specific or divided on their views about this. For example, for Buddhists, purposely hastening death is prohibited and the emphasis would be on trying to ease the patient's transition towards death and increasing their insight into suffering and its inevitable end. Encouraging a sick person to relax their grip on life or give up the will to live would not be seen as an act of compassion. The Islamic faith categorically forbids suicide, or assisted suicide; this would be an insult to Allah and people would not even be given burial rights http://en.wikipedia.org/wiki/Physician-assisted_suicide (*Physician-Assisted Suicide* 2008).

If patients felt that their concerns about an undignified or painful death were unfounded, then they might not feel the need to resort to assisted death as a way of maintaining control, even if this means travelling to another country. Therefore nurses need to take these end-of-life concerns very seriously in order to provide realistic reassurance about the help available at the end of people's lives.

> **THOUGHTS FOR YOUR PRACTICE**
>
> - How do you ensure that privacy is respected in relation to people within your practice environment?
> - Have there been times when privacy was compromised?
> - If this was the case, how could you have avoided this?
> - How do you maintain privacy of information when family, friends or carers are present?
> - How could you use quieter times in practice to try to get to know patients better and to actively seek their views?
> - Have you experienced times when a patient's death was undignified?
> - How could the patient's end-of-life care been more in keeping with their wishes?
> - What could you do to improve the quality of end-of-life care for patients in the future?

How do nurses perceive dignity in their practice?

CASE STUDY 3.3

Maisie was lying in bed wondering what life had become. She had been admitted to hospital from home the previous evening with acute retention of urine. She did not know why her bladder had stopped working, but apparently it had. A temporary catheter had been inserted to relieve the pressure and her discomfort and she had immediately felt better. However, now she was lying exposed from the waist down behind curtains in the middle of a busy ward. The reason she knew that the ward was busy was because she could see visitors, patients and nursing and medical staff bustling about through the gaps in the curtains. If she could see them, she knew that they must be able to see her, though most people tactfully kept their eyes averted.

Eventually, Kim, the nurse whom she had met for the first time on the ward round, opened the curtains and explained that she needed a more permanent catheter to solve the problem she had at the moment. Maisie had found the first catheterisation uncomfortable, but she was so relieved to feel better that she forgot about it almost immediately. However, now she could feel her anxiety building. She had not really understood any-thing that was said on the ward round. There were a lot of complicated words and nobody actually spoke to her and, if they looked at her, it was if they were looking at a specimen in a jar. She used to teach biology and she knew how some of the insects felt now, that she had kept as examples.

Kim did not seem to notice that Maisie now was totally exposed and although she was trying to explain what she was about to do, all Maisie could concentrate on were the people she could see through the gaps in the curtains. At that point a male doctor came through one of the gaps she was watching and asked Kim a question about another patient. Kim answered and he went out again, leaving a larger gap in the curtains. As Kim was about to start, another nurse came through the other gap in the curtains and asked for the drug keys. She detached them from Kim's belt and went out again leaving a larger gap in those curtains. Kim was obviously very keen to get this over and done with and Maisie said nothing, although Kim was obviously trying to put her at ease by asking her questions about herself and explaining her actions.

A male nurse then came through the first gap and said he was going on his break. As he left, increasing the size of gap in the curtains still more, Maisie burst into tears.

Discussion

Having discussed what dignity means to patients and clients, it is important to compare this with nurses' perceptions of dignity, and how this can be compromised within healthcare settings.

In the UK, Charlotte Potter, of the charity 'Help the Aged', emphasised the importance of establishing and maintaining dignity for patients as an issue of paramount importance. She says that 'nurses are key to ensuring dignity through care, but they do not work in a vacuum. If they do not receive appropriate support, patients will lose out'. (BBC News 2008). In response to this, Care Services Minister, Ivan Lewis, said, 'Nurses, like other NHS professionals, have a duty to treat patients with dignity at all times; however they also have a right to expect the necessary support and resources to make this possible.' (BBC News, 2008). This has been taken forward since then and respect and dignity are now one of the top priorities for the National Health Service (NHS), and will be high on the agenda for every hospital, care home and healthcare provider in the UK.

The NHS next stage review (DOH 2008) focused primarily on the importance of the patients' experience in terms of quality of care and quality of caring. This was seen as involving 'compassion, dignity and respect with which patients are treated' (p. 47). Patient satisfaction is now a major quality indicator and patient feedback needs to be actively sought and responded to by nurses. Patients who are not treated with dignity and respect will clearly be dissatisfied with the care they have received, and this is now seen as unacceptable. Nurses are now charged with leading practice, challenging unacceptable standards in practice and changing healthcare systems as necessary.

Kim might well have been very surprised by Maisie's tears, as she had her back to the gaps in the curtains and was focusing on the task in hand, communicating with Maisie as she felt appropriate at the time. To Kim, it perhaps felt normal to be interrupted in the middle of providing intimate care in the environment she was working in. However, Maisie was used to being treated with respect in her previous job and in life in general. She was certainly not used to lying exposed on a hospital bed, where people could see parts of her that should not be in the public domain. She accepted that Kim needed to access intimate areas of her body, but was very distressed by the fact that she was seen as an object that did not need to be respected by others who came into her bedspace, without even understanding her need for privacy, dignity or respect.

In order to promote dignity, Sturdy (2007) says that healthcare professionals need to 'protect those who are exposed to the alien, and often frightening, environment of care services' (p. 9). Kim needed to take an active role in protecting Maisie from having her privacy and dignity invaded in this alien environment in which she found herself. The culture of the ward needed to change so that nurses and other healthcare practitioners did not see it as acceptable to walk in on patients, who might be in a compromised state. In addition, the right equipment needed to be available to ensure that curtains fitted well, and perhaps that there was some indicator of the fact interruptions were to be avoided because of the nature of the care being undertaken. There have been examples of coloured pegs being used to close curtains, which give an indication of the importance of privacy. These would have helped in this situation, both by discouraging the interruptions in the first place, and by ensuring that there were no gaps in the curtains. Maisie's needs should have been seen as paramount and advanced planning could have avoided the need for handover of keys, or discussion of break times or another patient.

Ill-fitting curtains have been raised as a concern in terms of providing dignified care, but other examples are insufficient washing and toilet facilities, mixed sex wards, which can be distressing to both genders, and a lack of specialist lifting equipment, which can mean that people are being moved and handled inappropriately. In addition, some hoists can make people feel very vulnerable, particularly when they are used in a common area. This can be difficult to avoid, but a greater awareness by nursing staff of the importance of maintaining dignity wherever possible, and the recognition of how vulnerable they would feel if they were that patient, is an important cultural shift that needs to take place in many care environments. Kim certainly would not have wanted to be in Maisie's situation, and neither would any of the other healthcare professionals who interrupted her care.

Nurses in the UK have raised concerns about being unable to provide dignified care. In a poll of more than 2000 nurses, 8 out of 10 nurses said that they have left work distressed because they have been unable to treat patients with the dignity they deserve (BBC News 2008). Washing and privacy were cited as common issues of concern, as well as staff shortages and not being able to provide non-emergency patients will single-sex accommodation. One nurse said: 'Patients seem to be becoming numbers not people. I am having to fight against what the system wants in order to provide dignified care to my patients.' In total, 81% of those quizzed said they sometimes, or always, left their workplace feeling distressed or upset because they had not been able to give patients the kind of dignified care that they would want. In addition, 86% of the nurses polled said dignity should be a higher priority (Royal College of Nursing [RCN] 2008).

The RCN poll (RCN 2008) cited several issues that prevented dignified care:

➤ overcrowded wards;
➤ the layout of the clinical area;
➤ the curtains around the beds;
➤ noisy and disruptive environments;
➤ mixed sex wards.

Organisationally, these included:

➤ resources and staffing levels;
➤ overwhelming paperwork;
➤ targets and statistics;
➤ a lack of leadership on these issues.

Maisie would certainly have felt that her dignity was being compromised by the apparent busyness of the ward, the lack of effective curtaining and the mixed sex environment. She would have been unaware of the paperwork and the need to meet targets. However, she might have suspected that there were problems on this ward with staffing levels and a lack of leadership on issues that encouraged dignity. However, Kim and the other practitioners should have been aware of the impact of these factors and their influence on maintaining patient dignity. They also need to take a lead in challenging such practice and the organisational issues that can adversely affect the care given.

In the UK nurses are being given more responsibilities, particularly in relation to enhanced technology and the meeting of targets, which increases the amount of paperwork and computer orientated work that they need to do. In addition, enhanced roles can make nurses more task-orientated and focused on advanced skills. This can detract from them taking an active part in the fundamental care needs that people have, or at least supervising the quality of care that is required. Nurses need to take a lead in ensuring that patients' fundamental care needs are met. For example, patients might need to be encouraged to eat and helped with eating and drinking, if necessary. Systems need to be in place to ensure that nurses know when this is not happening. Coloured meal trays for those with particular nutritional needs have been used in some places to highlight when adequate nutrition is being compromised.

Having discussed some of the challenges that nurses face in ensuring that their patients or clients receive dignified care, it is important to develop strategies to support practitioners in their role in promoting dignity. The UK, Dignity Challenge and dignity champions (web site Dignity in Care) suggest various ways in which nurses can develop high quality services that respect people's dignity. These could include:

➤ having a zero tolerance of all forms of abuse;
➤ supporting people with the same respect you would want for yourself or a member of your family;
➤ treating each person as an individual by offering a personalised service;
➤ enabling people to maintain the maximum possible level of independence, choice and control;
➤ listening and supporting people to express their needs and wants;
➤ respecting people's right to privacy;
➤ ensuring that people feel able to complain without fear of retribution;
➤ engaging with family members and carers as care partners;
➤ assisting people to maintain confidence and a positive self-esteem;
➤ acting to alleviate people's loneliness and isolation.

By looking at this list of suggestions, it is easy to see the ways in which Maisie's dignity was not being protected, and the lack of leadership ensuring that dignity issues were seen as a priority.

Nurses need to understand and agree on what dignity means to patients and clients (Hunt 2008). They also need to develop influencing skills to make sure that the appropriate resources are available to allow dignified care to take place. Nurses also need to be assertive enough to take a zero tolerance approach to colleagues who treat patients disrespectfully. This could be in their role as practitioners or managers. Nurses need to be active listeners and use their verbal and non-verbal communication skills in order to really hear what patients actually need from the service they are providing.

THOUGHTS FOR YOUR PRACTICE

- How do you prevent interruptions to care that might compromise patients' dignity?
- How do you ensure that you have adequate resources and equipment in your practice environment to ensure that people have the best care possible in the circumstances?
- How would you take an active leadership role in challenging undignified practice?
- How could you start to influence changes in systems that do not promote patient dignity?
- How do you ensure that patients' fundamental care needs are met within your practice area?

KEY THEME TWO – RESPECT

CASE STUDY 3.4

Helen had been having a bad night shift on the Intensive Therapy Unit (ITU). The patient she was looking after, Omar, was deteriorating fast, despite the whole team's efforts to stabilise him. His young wife, Misha, was at his bedside, quietly crying, and she knew that their baby son was being looked after by his mother in the waiting room. It was so unfair. He had only been going to the late night shop to get some formula milk for the baby because they had run out. He was brutally attacked outside the shop by a young man who had been shouting racist insults as he carried on kicking and stamping on his head. Helen knew that Omar's head injury was too severe for him to survive and he had been unconscious since the attack. However, it had been established that he wanted his organs to be used for others, if such a situation arose. Helen listened as the transplant nurse discussed with Misha what organs could be retrieved, and she thought of the various people whose lives would be enhanced by the use of these organs.

In the next bed was a 50-year-old man who had been an alcoholic most of his life. His oesophageal varices were now starting to heal, but he was very jaundiced and was on the liver transplant list. When he had been admitted she had called him Mike, when apparently he was always called Mick, and he had been cross for her assumption that Mike was his name. She felt that he had overreacted because, after all, how was she to know his name? On the admission information it just said that his name was Michael. She knew that she should treat him with as much respect as any other patient, but she just could not respect his lifestyle choices. If Mick, or someone like him, received Omar's liver she felt it would be a betrayal of Omar's generosity and care for others. Omar had done nothing to deserve his untimely death; whereas Mick was lucky to have lived so long and his health problems were clearly of his own making. She knew that nobody would receive Omar's liver if they were continuing to drink, but she also knew of another patient who had stopped drinking for a year, had a transplant and then started drinking again and had died six months later. Helen felt this was such a waste of a precious organ.

She knew that she should be non-judgemental, but felt that she could identify more with younger people who had a lot to give and who had not made dubious life choices. The elderly, who had lived their lives, drunks, or those who had harmed others, she found much more difficult to nurse.

Discussion

It is clear that, while Helen obviously respects and values Omar, she has little time for Mick and his lifestyle choices. If respect is seen as treating others as you would want to be treated yourself – which is one of the basic tenets of compassion – she is finding this very difficult in her relationship with Mick. She is failing to acknowledge his worth or to respect and value him as an individual.

We have already discussed the importance of dignity and privacy, in terms of respect, but there are other elements of respect, which are of equal importance. Helen seemed surprised that Mick has responded badly to calling him by the wrong derivation of his name. Nurses are more informal nowadays and many patients are happier to be called by their first names. However, this is not always the case and people should be given a real choice about what they want to called, whether this is Mr Lewis, Michael, Mike or Mick. Helen made the assumption that he was happy to be called by his first name and then compounded this error of judgement by assuming that he would be called by a shortened version, and that shorter version was Mike. This negative start to their relationship might have been avoided if she had genuinely asked him what he liked to be called.

This is particularly true with older people who might feel much more comfortable being called by their last name. In fact, they might feel that it is disrespectful to be called by their first name by someone much younger than they are. Their identity is influenced by the person they are, but also by the generation they belong to. It is important to understand how our parents and grandparents might feel and to be careful with our use of language and ensure that we communicate in a respectful manner. Overall, a lack of formality can cause concern for older people but could reassure younger people. Informality and professionalism can coexist, but this has to be carefully managed.

It is apparent that Helen is not only judgemental, although she appreciates the need for her not to be in her role as a nurse, she is also stereotyping people as 'the elderly' and 'drunks'. Holt (2000) discusses this in relation to older people and suggests that the use of collective terms and group labelling such as 'elderly' imply the merging of millions of people whose lives have spanned four decades of human life and history into a single homogeneous group, which reveals a pitiful disregard for individual diversity. Holt continues by suggesting that 'there is a distinct need for care philosophies to embrace the heterogeneity of ageing and recognise each individual as an individual, not merely as a unit to be classified by age' (p. 56). Both these attitudes, which were displayed by Helen, form a real barrier to building a trusting relationship. These points will be discussed further in this chapter.

How do we build person-centred relationships?

CASE STUDY 3.5

Josh was very clear that he did not want to be here outside the school nurse's drop in room at all, but he knew he had to discuss this with someone. Whenever he had seen Becky around the school, she had always smiled and he felt that she was someone he would be able to talk to. So he took a deep breath and knocked on the door. When he heard her voice he almost bottled out and walked away. He made himself go in then sat on the chair at the side of her desk, facing her. Immediately she smiled and he felt himself relax a little. It was going to be difficult to know how to begin though.

He heard her say that it was nice to see him and she knew that, as a nurse, he could trust her to be confidential with whatever he told her. He started to try to say what he had come to talk about, but heard himself stammering. She said that it was good that he had come to see her now as she had plenty of time because nobody else was booked for the rest of the session. That helped him to realise that he did not need to say everything in a rush. She asked him what he most enjoyed doing and he heard himself say that he enjoyed rugby and wanted to do sports sciences at university. He was in his final year of school, so making choices about university courses seemed to be taking on a life of its own. As Becky started to ask about his rugby, Josh suddenly blurted out his innermost thoughts. He was a respected sportsman within the school and his macho image was well intact and he felt that he was constantly gently repelling advances from girls at the school. However, he had known for some time now that he was not interested in girls and he was pretty sure that he was gay.

Becky asked him what had made him think that he was gay initially, and he said that he found that he was attracted to the male form rather than the female pictures that his friends found attractive. He had not really taken this seriously at the time, but here he was, three years later, and he knew that his attraction for men was increasing rather than diminishing. He was really worried about how his parents and his friends would react, but firstly he was concerned about how Becky would react. Would she feel repulsed? Would she tell him it was just a phase? Would she laugh at him?

He didn't have the courage to look directly at her, but he heard her say gently that she knew how hard it was for him to tell anyone this and how glad she was that he had been brave enough to tell her. He looked up and saw the concern in her eyes and the steady way she met his gaze and knew that this was just the beginning of the discussions that he would have with her.

Discussion

This was a very traumatic situation for Josh. He had been keeping this very personal part of himself completely secret for some years, and now felt that it was time to discuss it with someone. He had seen Becky around the school and the fact that she had always smiled and seemed friendly had obviously made an impact on him. However, it was a new relationship that was being built at a time when he was trying to discuss very personal matters. His initial trust of her was as a nurse, who he saw as being a professional and who would respect him and his confidentiality.

This is borne out in a Canadian study by Trojan and Yonge (1993), who found that trusting, caring relationships were built on general trust, acceptance, respect and confidence in professional skills. They found that nurses were initially trusted because of their nursing qualification and expertise, but that the interaction that took place after the initial meeting was crucial to whether trust disappeared or developed. A nurse in the study says that:

> People are usually quite receptive as soon as you identify yourself, but it would depend a lot on how they interact with you on your initial visit whether or not the trust would stay there, or whether it is something that you are going to have to work on as the visits continue. (Trojan and Yonge 1993, p. 1905)

This study was carried out in relation to older people but it clearly is transferable to the building of any trusting relationship.

Becky had appeared to Josh as someone who was approachable and genuine and, therefore, he felt that he could trust her. Genuineness can be seen as being 'free from hypocrisy and dishonesty, actual, real, sincere or being yourself, honest and unpretentious' (Web site of The Free Dictionary). Becky exhibited all of these attributes, which drew Josh to her as someone he could confide in and trust. Rungapadiachy (1999) defines trust as being honest, open, sincere, supporting and dependable, genuine, warm and accepting. Again Becky demonstrated all of these traits.

Dowling (2006) says that respect is about building up an intimate relationship that involves a reciprocity and self-disclosure, getting to know the patient and allowing them to get to know the nurse as well. However, decreased hospital stays and resource reductions makes nursing more task orientated and this limits the opportunities for intimacy. Building relationships can be seen as a reasonable sacrifice in resource-limited organisations. Becky would have been busy, but she saw it as paramount that she gave the impression that her time was not limited in any way. Nurses need to try to develop this ability to seem as if they have sufficient time, regardless of their many demands, otherwise people will not disclose things to them and they will not see the true picture in relation to the individual's situation.

Trusting relationships allow people to disclose highly sensitive information that needs to be shared in order for optimal situations to develop. Difficult issues, such as abuse of older people, child protection, anger, domestic abuse, stress as a carer, inability to cope, fear of losing control or being hospitalised need to be understood in order to try to help those involved. These can only be divulged when there is trust between those involved and where there is privacy and confidentiality. However, as nurses we have a responsibility to ensure that patients and clients understand in advance the point at which confidentiality cannot be maintained. Illegal or damaging behaviour and abuse can not be kept confidential, because this involves the safety of others. However, other situations help the nurse to understand the stress that someone is feeling so that she can offer other solutions, which might prevent future harm.

For example, a man with paraplegia who was so terrified of being readmitted to hospital was unable to tell a community nurse who he trusted that he had deteriorating sacral sores. He did not tell her until the point where hospitalisation was inevitable and, actually, by that point he had septicaemia and was unlikely to survive. This could have been prevented, but the nurse involved had to conform to time-limited visits, which were less frequent than were needed, due to time constraints, an under-resourced team and frequent staff turnover. She was also new to the community and less experienced at identifying such matters. All of these issues can impact negatively on the ability to focus on therapeutic relationships and make building intimate relationships more difficult. Nurses need to be empowered to challenge resource constraints that make the building and maintaining of trusting relationships almost impossible. Holistic care and problem solving are severely compromised if resource constraints are negatively affecting trusting relationships.

Ensuring confidentiality can be very difficult within many practice environments. Breaches of confidentiality are not only unprofessional, but also severely damage trusting relationships with patients. Within a hospital setting, conversations behind curtains can be overheard. In any setting, a person could ask for someone else to be present, not realising the potential topics that could be covered during the ensuing conversation. Some communities are very close-knit and confidentiality can be more or less impossible to maintain; for example in schools, small villages and isolated communities where the nurse might live and work within the same community. The nurse may be totally confidential, but people might fear that she or he might not be. It is up to the nurse to raise confidentiality as an issue early in the relationship to reassure patients and clients that this is absolute, except in situations where there is a risk of harm to themselves or others, as discussed above.

THOUGHTS FOR YOUR PRACTICE

- How do you feel that you could give the impression of approachability to patients and clients before you actually build relationships with them?
- What do you do in your first contact with patients and clients to initiate a trusting relationship?
- How do you broach the subject of confidentiality at the start of your relationships?
- How do you ensure that your conversations are confidential?
- How do you balance resource constraints with building a trusting relationship with patients and clients?

Do we understand the importance of non-judgemental attitude?

CASE STUDY 3.6

Real life patient experience

Recently I had to have stitches removed from my arm that were needed after a self-inflicted injury.

I had to go to St Helens Walk-in Centre to have this done, as it was the weekend. I was not looking forward to it. Being somebody who self-injures, it meant I would have had to show my whole arm to this nurse and I wondered how they would react.

I don't know the name of the person I saw, but he asked me the dreaded question before I rolled my sleeve up: 'How did you do it?' I replied, 'Self-harm.' He encouraged me to roll my sleeve up.

He clearly picked up on my anxiety and reluctance to remove the dressing that would reveal yet more scars and the stitched wound. In a calm and gentle manner, he simply said, 'Go on, it's okay', and suddenly, I felt okay. Those few words just let me know that he wasn't going to ridicule me or treat me any differently.

He was gentle in removing the very awkward stitches and was clear in giving me information about aftercare (i.e. no perfumed products on it for at least three days, etc).

> This nurse could not have done a better job – not just at removing the stitches, but at making me feel at ease and not making me feel ashamed or guilty. There are nurses out there who could take a leaf out of his book and understand a little more about self-harm. In this instance, I was treated like a respected and valued human being – not some useless waste of space who didn't deserve the time of day because I'd hurt myself. (Web Site on Patient Opinion, ID 7908)

Discussion

In the example above, which comes from a patient opinion web site, the person involved is clearly highly anxious about having their stitches removed because of the fact that they are there because of a self-inflicted injury. The nurse involved is very sensitive and his non-judgemental approach is the most important part of the consultation. He makes the patient feel accepted and respected, rather than ashamed and guilty. People who exhibit behaviour that is not readily accepted by society; for example, self-harming, parasuicide, alcohol or drug misuse, are used to being treated with disdain and are very skilled at seeing when there is an underlying judgemental attitude, even if nothing is actually said to this effect.

Trojan and Yonge (1993) say that 'If a nurse cannot accept the client and their values, the development of a trusting nurse-patient relationship is impeded' (p. 1905). Without a non-judgemental attitude, a trusting relationship cannot develop. In a Welsh study, De Raeve (2002) says that 'trust between people as individuals may emerge and increase, as people become more revealed and known to each other' (p. 161). In Case study 3.4, Helen would have been unable to build a trusting relationship with Mick because her judgemental attitude would have been in the way. However, in Case studies 3.5 and 3.6, it is clearly apparent that neither person was being judged by the nurses involved.

An English study written by Repper, Ford and Cooke (1994), concerning mental health clients, also emphasises the importance of a non-judgemental attitude in building a trusting relationship. They say that trust needs to develop in order for clients to feel able to show their vulnerability. Clients had to feel that they could expose these parts of themselves in the safe and sure knowledge that they would not be judged, or the information used to refer them elsewhere or to discharge them from care.

It is important that nurses really change their biases and prejudices so that they can practise in a non-judgemental manner. For example, in a community setting Trojan and Yonge (1993) talk about the importance of acceptance and non-judgemental attitude 'as one nurse stated "my feeling is that I am a guest in their homes. If I can't accept what they have got in their homes, their living conditions, then that is my problem, not their problem"' (p. 1905).

Cultural norms and values can play a part in whether nurses can accept a person or patient's situation or lifestyle. In a study of Egyptian caregivers, Boggatz and Dassen (2006), found that carers had to overcome fear, disgust, repetition and sexual taboo in their care of older people. They had to challenge their traditional values to care for their patients in the Egyptian care home in which they worked.

McHarg (2008) reports from the perspective of a friend on the care of a patient in hospital shortly before his death. The friend was a man with advanced Alzheimer's disease and his friend says:

> The condition was irreversible; he'd lost his memory and could be difficult. But the nurses always treated him as the gentleman he had been, not the awkward child he sometimes became. They never laughed at him. They allowed him his dignity. The Max I knew would have appreciated that. (p. 14)

The patient in this situation was never mocked or denigrated. He was respected in his changed circumstances, and that would have been important not only to him, but to his friends and relatives.

If nurses do not get this right then the impact on care is clearly inadequate and damaging.

> Nurses say that patients become distressed and confused if they are not treated with respect and if clinicians fail to communicate properly with them, which means the onus is on nurses to ensure their interpersonal skills are polished. Patients who feel they are not receiving the right levels of service may become angry and emotional . . . If you don't treat them right, they may become aggressive. (Staines 2008, p. 15)

This is understandable as nobody would want to be treated without dignity and respect. The person in Case study 3.6, who had self-harmed, might well have reacted in this way as they were expecting the staff to have a negative attitude. People who are continually treated without respect by practitioners who 'judge' them become angry or disempowered as a result, and can be reluctant to seek help.

THOUGHTS FOR YOUR PRACTICE

- Have you ever judged somebody, based purely on their appearance, life choices or circumstances?
- In your practice, how can you challenge these attitudes in yourself and others?
- Are you aware of your own biases and prejudice?
- How do you stop these impacting on your role as a nurse?

SUMMARY – LINKS TO COMPASSION AND CARING

We do not believe that compassionate care can exist without dignity and respect being central to the relationship between nurse and patient or client. Dignity has to be considered primarily from the patient's or client's perspective. People need to be listened to and understood in terms of what is important to them. They want to be treated as individuals, as we would ourselves. They want their privacy to be respected and time to build relationships with nursing staff. Nurses can find it difficult to meet these needs in the current healthcare environment, with a potential focus on targets rather than quality of care. Nurses need to take a lead in challenging undignified care in themselves and others, and in challenging systems that compromise their ability to provide dignified care.

The importance of trust in building respectful relationships cannot be underestimated. People need to feel that their confidentiality is not being compromised and that their care is individualised and based around their specific circumstances. They also need to feel that they are accepted and valued, regardless of their life situation or lifestyle choices. Without these important components of respect and dignity, compassionate care is absent.

> When dignity and respect are absent from care, people feel devalued, lack control and comfort. They may also lack confidence, be unable to make decisions for themselves, and feel humiliated, embarrassed and ashamed. Providing dignity in care centres on three integral aspects: respect, compassion and sensitivity. In practice this means:
> **Respecting** patients' and clients' diversity and cultural needs; their privacy – including protecting it as much as possible in large, open-plan hospital wards; and the decisions they make;
> Being **compassionate** when a patient or client and/or their relatives

need emotional support, rather than just delivering technical nursing care;

Demonstrating **sensitivity** to patients' and clients' needs, ensuring their comfort' (Royal College of Nursing 2008).

Peter Carter, general secretary of the RCN, says, 'Dignity should not be an after-thought or an optional extra. Each and every patient – whether they are in a hospital, a GP's surgery, in the community or in a care home – deserves to be treated with dignity and respect' (BBC News 2008).

In addition, the Chief Nursing Officer for England, Christine Beasley, says, 'I believe strongly that dignity, respect, care and compassion are at the heart of good nursing care whenever and wherever it takes place' (BBC News 2008).

REFERENCES

BBC News (2008) *Nurses Raise Dignity Concerns*. Available at: http://news.bbc.co.uk/1/hi/health/7363525.stm (accessed 27 April 2008).

Boggatz T, Dassen T. Learning the meaning of care: a case study in a geriatric home in Upper Egypt. *J Transcult Nurs*. 2006; **17**(2): 155–63.

Carter H, MacLeod R, Brander P, *et al.* Living with a terminal illness: patients' priorities. *J Adv Nurs*. 2004; **45**(6): 611–20.

Charles-Edwards I, Brotchie J. Privacy: what does it mean for children's nurses? *Paediatric Nursing*. 2005; **17**(5): 36–43.

De Raeve L. Trust and trustworthiness in nurse-patient relationships. *Nursing Philosophy*. 2002; **3**(2): 152–62.

Department of Health. *High Quality Care for All: NHS next stage review final report*. Cm 7432. London: Department of Health; 2008.

Dowling M. The sociology of intimacy in the nurse-patient relationship. *Nursing Standard*. 2006; **20**(23): 48–54.

Holt I. Age is not a barrier to individuality. *Br J Community Nurs*. 2000; **(5)**2: 56.

Hunt L. Dignity should rage across every ward. *Nurs Times*. 2008; **104**(26): 18–19.

Lewis I. Speech by Ivan Lewis MP, Parliamentary Undersecretary of State for Care Services. *Dignity in Care Campaign Launch*. 14 November 2006. Available at: www.dh.gov.uk/en/News/Speeches/DH_065414 (accessed 27 February 2008).

McHarg L. Dignity is vital in older people's care. *Nurs Times*. 2008; **104**(4): 14.

Merriam-Webster. *Online Dictionary*. Available at: www.merriam-webster.com/dictionary/sensitivity (accessed 3 April 2008).

Oregon State Web site. *Death with Dignity Act* (1997). Available at: www.oregon.gov/DHS/ph/pas/docs/year10.pdf (accessed 16 July 2008).

Parkinson M. Britain's shame. *Daily Mail*. 29 May 2008; p. 14.

Physician-Assisted Suicide. Available at: http://en.wikipedia.org/wiki/Physician-assisted_suicide (accessed 13 May 2008).

Repper J, Ford R, Cooke A. How can nurses build trusting relationships with people who have severe and long-term mental health problems? Experiences of case managers and their clients. *J Adv Nurs.* 1994; **19**(6): 1096–104.

Royal College of Nursing. Available at: www.rcn.org.uk/newsevents/campaigns/dignity/the_rcns_dignity_survey (accessed 17 July 2008).

Rungapadiachy D. *Interpersonal Communication and Psychology for Healthcare Professionals.* Oxford: Butterworth Heinemann; 1999.

Shotton L, Seedhouse D. Practical dignity in caring. *Nurs Ethics.* 1998; **5**(3): 246–55.

Staines R. Is patient power good for nurses? *Nurs Times.* 2008; **104**(13): 13–16.

Sturdy D. Indignity in care: are you responsible? *Nurs Older People.* 2007; **19**(9): 9.

Trojan L, Yonge O. Developing trusting, caring relationships: home care nurses and elderly clients. *J Adv Nurs.* 1993; **18**(12): 1903–10.

Walsh K, Kowanko I. Nurses and patients' perceptions of dignity. *Int J Nurs Pract.* 2002; **8**(3): 143–51.

www.dignityincare.org.uk

www.patientopinion.org.uk/opinion.aspx?opinionID=7908

www.thefreedictionary.com/genuineness

CHAPTER 4

Listening and responding

Overview of the chapter

Key theme one – listening
- Case study
- Discussion
- Why is it essential to ensure that patients and clients have time to talk?
- Case study
- Discussion
- Thoughts for your practice
- Do we actually hear what patients and clients are telling us?
- Case study
- Discussion
- Thoughts for your practice

Key theme two – responding
- Case study
- Discussion
- How do we ensure that we respond appropriately to patient/client concerns?
- Case study
- Discussion
- Thoughts for your practice
- Do we keep our focus on the patient while carrying out nursing tasks?
- Case study
- Discussion
- Thoughts for your practice
- Summary – links to compassion and caring
- References

OVERVIEW OF THE CHAPTER

Through our discussions so far, it will be apparent how vitally important effective listening and appropriate responding are to patients and clients and that these skills have to be central to compassionate nursing care. Therefore, this chapter will concentrate on listening skills in terms of helping people to talk and providing the right opportunities for them to do so. Barriers to effective listening will be discussed and how these relate to the importance of actually hearing what people are saying, or not saying, to us. We need to listen to patients' experiences and views in order to provide more opportunities to be more person-centred in our practice.

Having listened to what people have to say, we need to respond appropriately by focusing on what the patient or client actually needs, as opposed to just the tasks that need to be carried out from the nursing perspective.

Discussing these points in relation to listening and responding will, we hope, give you the chance to revisit your own nursing care in relation to these important areas and take practice forward as appropriate.

KEY THEME ONE – LISTENING

CASE STUDY 4.1

There was no denying that George was in pain. His hip replacement the day before had gone smoothly enough and he was relieved that the surgery was over. However, despite repeated requests for analgesia, he was still lying in bed having been given nothing to ease the pain. Pain always made him irritable and now two nurses were at his bedside saying they 'wanted to freshen him up and make him comfortable'. The only comfort he wanted at the moment was something to help the pain and the thought of being moved around without this filled him with dread. He tried to express this as strongly as he could without being critical. One of nurses replied that the drug round would be starting soon and he would be able to have something then. Despite several attempts it seemed impossible to actually get her to define how soon 'soon' would be. He explained that he would really rather prefer to let this work before he was moved about, but the other nurse just said, 'It won't take long', as if that was the answer that solved everything.

So there he was lying down and being manhandled by both of them while he gritted his teeth to counter the increased pain he was feeling.

They were talking to each other about a night out they'd had the night before and he felt like he may as well be just a sack of potatoes for all the notice they were taking of him. He was glad that they had enjoyed their free time, but they were not even communicating with him at all; not even to tell him what they were going to do next.

He was feeling desperate and quite faint from the increasing pain when another nurse came behind the curtains. She seemed to immediately sense his discomfort and distress and moved to his side and held his hand. The other nurses appeared to be more junior because their chatting about their social lives stopped immediately. The new nurse spoke to him quietly and gently and asked him how bad the pain was, as if the fact that he was in pain was not in dispute. She asked him which position he was most comfortable in and then made sure he was in that position. She then explained that she would give him an injection and leave him to rest while it took effect and then they would come back to finish helping him wash. He could have cried with relief that she had seemed to understand his distress even though she had not been there to hear him express his need for analgesia a few minutes earlier. He concluded that this was the sign of an expert and compassionate nurse.

Discussion

George had been trying to explain that his hip pain was increasing and that he needed some analgesia. However, he was also trying to explain that he really needed this before he was moved and before any planned nursing tasks were going to be carried out. The nurses were clearly not hearing what he was actually saying; therefore they were not actually listening. Rungapadiachy (1999) says that 'listening can be defined as the art of capturing the true essence of the sender's message' (p. 214). Wolvin and Coakley (1996) say that 'therapeutic listening involves empathy, which is feeling and thinking with another person' (p. 279). In this case, the nurses were clearly not taking on board George's message and they were not being empathetic in hearing what he was actually saying.

Harteveldt (2008) highlights the importance of listening as a way of improving patient well-being. The ability to communicate is the key. It does not always require long conversations, but choosing the appropriate words or simply offering a listening ear is enough. This can radiate a sense of empathy and a feeling of caring and can relieve a patient's stress. We can be too focused on targets, as these nurses were in wanting to get the task of washing George over as quickly as possible.

> We all have to remember that whatever a person's medical, mental or physical disability, they are still human beings . . . nursing and care staff should, wherever possible, get to know the client as an individual and find out how best to communicate with them in a manner that does not patronise. (Bordiak 2008, p. 10)

The more senior nurse took just a few minutes to do just this.

In an American article, Vora and Vora (2008) discuss different approaches to listening:

➤ **discriminative listening** – listening to distinguish among auditory and visual stimuli;

➤ **comprehensive listening** – listening to comprehend and retain information;

➤ **therapeutic listening** – listening for the purpose of helping another person, and to learn when to ask questions, when to stimulate further discussion, and when, if ever, to give advice;

➤ **critical listening** – listening to assess and evaluate what one comprehends (pp. 66–7).

The first two nurses did not even appear to use discriminative listening; however, the senior nurse was able not only to use auditory and visual stimuli to assess George's pain levels, but also was then able to retain this information to use it for therapeutic purposes. Her critical listening skills enabled her to change the care that was given, based on her interpretation of what she was seeing and hearing. As a result, George felt genuinely nurtured and cared about, because he was genuinely being listened to.

In a Canadian paper, Jonas-Simpson, *et al.* (2006) identified various themes in relation to being listened to:

➤ **nurturing contentment** – if someone feels listened to they feel good, gratified, unburdened, satisfied, and cared about;

➤ **vital genuine connections** – if someone feels listened to, the relationship between the nurse and the patient is strengthened;

➤ **deference triumphs mediocrity** – the 'reality that respect and the benefits of being listened to are more poignant than those of disregard in institutions where mediocrity or neutrality is expected' (p. 51).

Therefore, people who are being cared for in an institution where they do not expect to be listened to tend to feel there is no point in saying anything, as nobody listens to them. It is important for all of us to feel appreciated, and people can tell when they, or others, are genuinely being listened to. Disregard, and being treated with indifference when not being listened to, cause frustration and can make a person feel insignificant. If people's wishes are respected, taken seriously and deferred to, they are more likely to feel listened to. It causes annoyance if there is no response to a request or a suggestion. If you are listened to you can feel you want to do things and achieve things, rather than feeing low and demotivated.

As a patient says on a patient opinion web site:

> In my opinion, neither my GP nor the ENT consultant listened to my story and so did not treat my ear appropriately. They ignored my observations that the symptoms would go dormant and then return. As a result I have suffered far more than necessary and a lot of NHS time and money has been wasted unnecessarily. I feel that the moral for the medical profession is to follow the elementary rule of listening to the patient. (Web Site on Patient Opinion, ID 7838)

George could have started to feel demotivated, devalued and worthless if the way the first two nurses treated him had continued, particularly if he had been in this environment for an extended period of time. Apart from the fact that the nurses were missing an opportunity to build a positive relationship with him, and assess his health status, they were having a negative impact on his physical and psychological well-being.

Why is it essential to ensure that patients and clients have time to talk?

CASE STUDY 4.2

Sugandh was very worried. Her daughter Annesha had been admitted again with a chest infection, which was a pretty common occurrence for her, unfortunately. The condition, which had resulted in her learning disability, also left her very vulnerable physically to frequent hospital admissions. Therefore, Sugandh was highly sensitive to the impression nursing staff gave on Annesha's admissions to hospital. She found that sometimes nurses genuinely listened to what she was saying about Annesha's specific needs, and in those cases the response to those needs seemed to permeate through the whole team and Annesha was treated as the 'special' child that she was. On other occasions she would feel that the admitting nurse was treating her as someone to be tolerated, but really they did not need to know all this detail. Those were the times when she felt that she needed to be with Annesha for as much time as she could manage, so that she did not deteriorate and withdraw during her time in hospital.

On this occasion, the nurse, who had introduced herself as Liz, seemed busy and distracted. Sugandh tried to explain that Annesha needed to have her soft toy around her to cuddle, as it gave her comfort and also that she found music soothing and had her MP3 player with earphones, which she liked to listen to most of the time. However, she could see that Liz was bustling around, taking Annesha's temperature and filling in paperwork and was not even making eye contact with Sugandh. Liz seemed to be in a hurry and certainly did not appear to want to listen to things that were so important to her daughter. The emphasis seemed to be on getting things done and not listening to her very real concerns about Annesha's particular needs while she was in hospital

Sugandh knew that hearing what she had to say, as Annesha could not say for herself, was an important part of the assessment process. Was Liz even aware of this? She knew that she would not feel safe in leaving Annesha here for extended times, without her, and she had two other children at home, one of whom also had special needs. She could feel her anxiety levels rising and she felt that she was being dismissed as an overprotective mother. The fact that Liz was not even listening to her made her feel tearful, tired and misunderstood.

Discussion

In Case study 4.2, Sugandh was clearly not feeling listened to. She was not being given time to express her fears and convey her knowledge of her daughter to those who would be caring for her. She was absolutely correct that Liz needed to hear about her daughter as this is part of the holistic assessment process. There should be adequate time to listen to the patient, client or carer on first meeting them. The carer's perspective is a particularly important part of the assessment process, when an individual cannot express their own needs or act as their own advocate. This example is about a girl with a learning disability, but the same would be true if someone who could not talk due to having suffered a stroke, or someone with advanced dementia, was being admitted. Active listening, to reassure Sugandh that she was being heard, would have enabled a partnership to be developed, and potentially for shared and empowered decision making to take place. This is possible whatever the patient's or client's situation.

McCabe (2004), in an Irish paper, talks about the importance of attending behaviour, in terms of accessibility and readiness to listen, which is clearly evident through non-verbal communication. The importance of giving time and being there, being open and honest in our communication and being genuine are so important in any interaction with clients and patients. Active listening is a key part of this process. However, this is a complex process. What the patient or client says might not be what they actually mean, and what the nurse hears might not be translated into what she understands (Ewles and Simnett 2003). There is a strong potential for misunderstanding on both parts and this is a real barrier to effective communication and compassionate care.

The importance of giving people time to talk cannot be overestimated. Many people need to be given help in order to talk about issues that are personal to them. Many people need to be encouraged to give their views and perceptions and a specific invitation to do so can help in this process. Sugandh was never offered this opportunity to give her views, although she tried to play an active part in the assessment process. She was certainly never invited to talk about Annesha's needs, let alone her own needs as a carer. Liz did not pay sufficient attention to what Sugandh was saying, and verbal and non-verbal channels of communication were blocked. Sugandh should have been encouraged to explain her concerns as there was probably a great deal that was left unsaid. Nurses need to use a variety of techniques to reinforce the fact that they are listening. These could include verbal interventions like 'Mmm, go on', or nodding or showing understanding by saying something like 'so you are saying . . .' The use of paraphrasing, summarising and reflecting meanings and feelings, checking for accuracy and understanding by restating what Sugandh was saying in different words, could have been be useful. In addition, mirroring back the feelings that she was expressing by saying something like 'You are worried about Annesha while she is in hospital because . . .' would have reassured Sugandh that she was not only being listened to, but heard. Demonstrating understanding of Sugandh's perspective and listening to not only what she was saying, but also how she was saying it, would have demonstrated active listening and empathetic understanding, which relies heavily on having time to talk. Vora and Vora (2008) emphasise the importance of actively listening and giving people time to talk, particularly when people are nearing the end of their lives. This provides comfort, which in itself can be a form of healing.

The use of appropriate questions to help someone to talk can be central to finding out what their problems and needs are. The use of open-ended questions is often seen as giving people maximum opportunity to express their thoughts, and in most cases this is true and will encourage a full response and a broader consideration of relevant issues. However, when someone is underconfident or is finding it difficult to express themselves, open questions can make them feel inhibited and responses can become limited. For example, a young person might find it easier to respond to closed questions with minimal eye contact if they are finding the conversation embarrassing. The use of closed questions, or gradually funnelled questions, can help to clarify details; for example, 'What do you find tends to soothe Annesha?' followed by 'When is it most helpful for Annesha to listen to her music?' Nurses need to be skilled and sensitive to know what sort of questioning would be most helpful in which circumstances. Questions that can appear detailed, caring and reassuring in some cases can be intrusive and threatening in others.

In complete contrast to active listening, Liz was letting barriers get in the way of her finding out what her new patient's needs actually were, and therefore her assessment would be incomplete. She was missing out on the opportunity to hear about Annesha from the person who knew her best, and was not building a relationship with Sugandh or Annesha. She was short of time and probably thought it was quicker – but quicker for whom, because in the end this insight would have proved invaluable and would save time trying to soothe Annesha when the nursing team would have no idea of what actually comforted her. If someone who cannot speak easily, such as an individual who has suffered a stroke, has cerebral palsy, or even has a stammer is not given adequate time to express themselves, or someone finishes off their sentences to try to rush what is being said, the patient will start to feel there is no point in speaking at all. The same would be true if an individual was distracted and confused; time pressures and being made to feel rushed would only make the situation worse. It is also important not to make assumptions about people based on their facial expressions; for example, with someone who has Parkinson's disease or myasthenia gravis. It would be easy to make assumptions that the 'mask-like' facial expression portrays the person's personality.

Stuart and Knott (2008) have identified various behaviours that block communication. These include:

➤ **normalising** – which belittles their experiences (e.g. 'Everyone feels that way after . . .');
➤ **false reassurance** – 'I'm sure the scan will show everything is fine';
➤ **leading questions** – which influences the response (e.g. 'You seem better today, don't you?');
➤ **deferring** – uncomfortable questions that a patient raises with a nurse should not be referred to a colleague to answer because this tends to

block the conversation. The patient has trusted that specific nurse and raised the issue with him/her and that trust should be respected. The question should be answered by them;

➤ **multiple questions** – it can appear as if the nurse is not interested in the answers because two or more questions have been asked at once;

➤ **platitudes** – the idea might be to cheer someone up, but they can make things worse (e.g. 'It can't be that bad, give me a smile') (p. 26).

Liz was more concerned with getting the admission process completed as quickly as possible, which was a barrier to communication in its own right. Other barriers to active listening can be:

➤ preoccupation with what you want to say next;
➤ self-consciousness;
➤ stress;
➤ anxiety;
➤ poor attention;
➤ misinterpretation;
➤ rehearsing responses.

Liz was not hampered in her listening skills by these factors because she had never engaged in the process of active listening concerning Annesha's needs or what Sugandh was trying to say to her. However, nurses need to be aware of these additional barriers to effective listening and communication.

THOUGHTS FOR YOUR PRACTICE

- Are you ever concerned that you do not have sufficient time to actively listen to your patients and clients during the assessment process?
- How could you try to enhance your ability to listen to what patients, carers and clients have to say in your interactions with them?
- Do you give people the opportunity to talk about their concerns?
- What approaches do you use to encourage people to talk?
- What sort of questions do you use in your practice, and are they always the most appropriate questions to ask?
- What barriers do you think there are in your practice area that might prevent you actively listening to your patients and clients?

Do we actually hear what patients and clients are telling us?

CASE STUDY 4.3

Tanya was visiting Mary for the first time. Her role as a community mental health nurse in the older person team meant that she visited many people who had increasing memory loss and who might have limited sensory faculties. She was so aware of how confusing life must seem for them and it was so important to get a sense of who they actually were, even if they could not tell her themselves. She always made time to talk to relatives who could give her information about a person's life history and interests. She also made sure that she built in sufficient time to start to get to know the person themselves and tried to get them to talk about themselves.

Mary had obviously had a very difficult life. She was the oldest of seven children and her mother had died young, leaving Mary to look after the younger children while her father worked to keep the family with only just enough food to keep them from starvation. She had been very happily married to her husband, Bill, but he had also died at a young age from a mining accident, leaving her to bring up a young family. All this she gleaned from Mary's daughter Julie. When Tanya asked what Mary enjoyed in life, Julie replied that she had always enjoyed music and loved animals and flowers.

When Tanya spoke to Mary, Mary looked at her with empty eyes. Gradually Tanya started to get some response from her and she started to respond to questions about her children and Bill. It was clear that she was not able to clearly differentiate between what was happening in the present day and what had happened in the past, but she was starting to talk. Tanya asked Julie if they had any pets and Julie replied that they had a guinea pig, who loved to be held. Tanya asked Julie if she could bring the guinea pig to her and also asked if there were any flowers in the garden. Julie was a keen gardener and Tanya asked her to bring a flower that was as fragrant as possible.

When Julie brought the guinea pig Tanya held it and asked Mary if she would like to stroke it. Mary seemed pleased with the idea, so Tanya guided Mary's hand so that she could stroke the soft fur. Tanya could see Mary start to relax as she stroked the pet. Tanya then said that there was a beautiful rose that Mary might like to smell. Mary had a significant amount of visual loss, but she breathed in deeply the fragrance of the flower. She asked what colour it was and when Tanya said that it was bright red, Mary started to talk about some bright red roses that Bill used to grow on his allotment. He always brought them home for her on her birthday.

Mary, by now, seemed to be totally at ease with Tanya and they started to talk about music she enjoyed. Mary said that she used to love Glenn Miller's music and although she had some old records, she had nothing to play them on any more. Just then Jed, her grandson, walked in and said that he had the equipment to transfer some of her old records onto his MP3 player and he would lend Mary his to listen to her favourite music, as she obviously missed it so much.

Overall Tanya thought that the visit had gone well. She had managed to engage Mary's senses, despite her vision loss, and the rest of the family were obviously highly motivated towards helping Mary to get as much out of life as possible. It was clear they were a loving family and through the narratives of both Julie and Mary she felt that she had started to get to know Mary, and could therefore think of ways to enhance her quality of life as much as possible.

Discussion

Tanya was clearly placing a great deal of importance on hearing what Mary was actually saying. She was using this information to build up a picture of who Mary actually was. Although she asked Julie for her help in trying to get to know her mother, she was clearly seeing Mary as a person in her own right and she wanted to try to gain information from her too. She could use this information to try to stimulate Mary's senses through touch, sound and smell.

Hawkins and Lindsay (2006) highlight the importance of listening to the patient's story because what is revealed 'gives it a deeper and clearer meaning for the teller especially if the telling is assisted by skilled listening' (p. S6). By doing so, nurses can raise an individual's self-esteem and genuinely enhance their life experiences, which can have the effect of helping them to feel more empowered to take more control over their life. 'The use of patient narratives cannot be overestimated as these stories demonstrate that the patient does not stand alone, but rather is part of a web of influences that includes the nurses and other patients' (p. S12). 'Stories can only be told when people have time to talk and listeners have sufficient time to hear: the richer the narrative, the more time is needed' (p. S14). This is very apparent in Mary's situation. She was not standing alone; her family and Tanya were standing with her. However, they all needed to give Mary enough time to relax and express herself, and genuinely want to hear what she was saying, in order for Tanya to be able to help them enhance Mary's quality of life.

It is important to listen and hear what is said in order to work in partnership to determine what needs to be achieved. This helps to build up a trusting relationship where individuals feel safe to divulge personal information that can be used as part of the assessment process to identify what the patient expects and needs. The outcome of the resulting partnership could be a jointly conceived plan for the way forward. This can be based more on the client's or patient's priorities and may not match the agenda that the nurse had in mind at the beginning of the consultation. To ensure that the individual's priorities, fears and concerns are central to the conversation, these need to be expressed as early as possible, otherwise they will not be capable of listening, or taking an active part in their future care because the focus is not on their agenda. Tanya clearly focused on Mary's interests during her first visit and she was able to find out information that would be useful for the future planning of her care.

Tanya was also skilled in creating an environment that minimised the natural power imbalance that can exist between a healthcare professional and a patient or client. By not interrupting, Tanya did not want to distract Mary from the picture she was painting of herself. She gave Mary her undivided attention and the impression that she had plenty of time.

THOUGHTS FOR YOUR PRACTICE

- Do you give your patients sufficient time to talk?
- Do you find that you can use information in their narratives to find ways to enhance their quality of life?
- Can you think of ways in which you can use these skills more in your practice?
- Can you think of examples from your practice where you have been able to stimulate different senses in your patients to enhance their care?
- How do you ensure that patients and clients have the opportunity to raise their fears and concerns at an early stage in your contact with them?

KEY THEME TWO – RESPONDING

CASE STUDY 4.4

Ben was not frightened though he knew that his parents were. He knew they thought that he did not understand what death actually was, but he understood that it was permanent and that there was no going back once death was inevitable. When his parents visited he could tell they were trying to be brave in front of him, but he could see from their red rimmed eyes and forced smiles that it was becoming increasingly difficult.

From his own point of view, he was so tired and just wanted to sleep, even if that sleep never ended. He just could not force himself to fight any more, but did not know how to tell his parents that. He felt that he owed it to them to carry on struggling to survive because they loved him so much and did not want to let him go.

As soon as Mark walked into the room, he could see the change in Ben. Mark had nursed Ben every time he had come into the children's hospice and he knew him well. He could see the exhaustion and desperation in his eyes today. Ben was not typical of most eight-year-olds, but then he had not lived the same life as most eight-year-olds. The degenerative neurological condition that he had been diagnosed with at 18 months of age had robbed him of a 'normal' childhood. He had been unable to climb trees, dash around on his bike or run and walk as other children did. He had not been able to become increasingly independent as he got older – in fact quite the reverse: he became increasingly dependent as the cruel condition took its course.

Mark asked Ben what was worrying him as he could see that something was up. Ben explained how tired he felt and how fed up he was with all the tubes and the painful interventions that were necessary, more and more frequently, to keep him alive. He wanted to stop fighting now, he knew the end was near however hard he fought, and he was very upset about the grief that his parents and older sister were about to face. He did not know how to tell them that he really could not do it anymore and he wanted to let go of life.

Mark found the conversation very hard, as he had grown to really care about this brave and funny boy, who always wanted to race others in his wheelchair, whether they were also in wheelchairs or on foot. He had a real zest for life and he would always be fondly remembered by so many people. However, Mark knew that Ben was right – he was nearing the end of his life. Mark felt that everyone should have some control over the end of their lives when they were suffering from a life-limiting condition. Why should Ben be any different because he was only eight years old?

Ben's parents were about to arrive and Mark asked Ben what he wanted to do. Ben said that he did not think that he could cope with telling his parents himself without someone else there to care for them if they became very distressed.

Mark said that he would be there while Ben talked to them, if that was what he wanted. He also said that somehow, he knew that they would understand. They knew more than anyone else how hard life had been for Ben and would not want him to suffer more than was necessary. The hospice was well equipped to help the whole family during this traumatic and terrible time. If these were Ben's wishes then support would be there for him, his sister and his family, together and separately.

Discussion

In his seminal work, Egan (1977) says that 'the ultimate proof of good listening is good responding' (p. 137). Rungapadiachy (1999) agrees with this and says that 'listening without responding is seen as hollow listening' (p. 221) and that 'responding can be defined as the art of giving appropriate feedback to the message received. Obviously responding would involve the processes of listening and attending.' (p. 221).

Egan (1977) says:

> Responding lies at the heart of the process of interpersonal communication and if one is to communicate effectively, then one has to master the skills of responding with accurate understanding. Responding with understanding is the recipe for caring. Responding with understanding suggests that the listener
> > listens carefully to the client's total message;
> > recognises the speaker's feeling and the behaviours which gave rise to these feelings;
> > demonstrates empathic understanding' (p. 221).

Mark clearly not only listened to and heard Ben's deep concerns, but he understood the total message he was trying to express, and what had given rise to these feelings. He also demonstrated clear empathy in his response to Ben's plea for support. Therefore, Mark clearly demonstrated how skilled he was in responding appropriately to Ben with compassion and caring in a very distressing situation.

This is a really good example of a skilled response to feedback being part of an informed approach to decision making, where Ben has expressed a need to choose his own destiny. He was well aware of relevant information and Mark was confident that Ben understood the implications of his decision. This contrasts strongly with the parental or paternalistic approach to care, which keeps the health professional as the sole decision maker. In the shared treatment decision-making model, advocated in an American/Canadian study, patients and clinicians are partners who participate fully in the process (Montori, Gafni and Charles 2006). This approach appeared to be helpful to all involved in the process.

How do we ensure that we respond appropriately to patient/client concerns?

CASE STUDY 4.5

Mike was lying awake in his bed on the surgical ward following his operation and he was watching the minutes on the clock going past interminably slowly. Why do nights always pass so slowly and seem so lonely when you are worried about something? Everyone around him seemed to be sleeping peacefully and although he could not say he was actually in pain, he certainly felt as if he was becoming more distressed and he could feel his anxiety levels increasing with every passing minute.

Abdul had been keeping an eye on Mike throughout the shift. Mike had returned from surgery for a prostatectomy for cancer of the prostate. Mike was 42 years old and the cancer was not confined to the prostate itself, and Abdul knew that the prognosis was not very good. Abdul also knew that Mike knew this too, and the surgeon had spoken to him when he returned to the ward following surgery. Abdul had seen Mike's wife and two small children leaving when he came on duty that evening and he also knew that the diagnosis had only been made last week.

Abdul could not imagine how he would deal with such a terrible situation, and now that the ward had quietened down a little he could see that Mike was still lying awake looking at the clock. He went over to him and sat down on the chair by Mike's bed. He hoped this would give the impression that Abdul had time to talk because despite the fact that the ward was busy, he felt that Mike was the priority at the moment.

Mike looked at him with eyes that were full of despair. Abdul decided that there was no point in hedging around the subject – that would just increase Mike's distress. He needed to show that he was with him in his time of despair. He said that it must have been such a shock to be told about the prostate cancer the week before. Mike responded immediately, saying that he was so young, he had a young family and that he knew that his prognosis was not good. He asked what he could have done to have prostate cancer so young. Abdul nodded and replied that life is not always fair – he had seen that so many times over his nursing career. He also said that nobody is immune, we could all of us be diagnosed with something potentially life threatening. He said that he was a similar age to Mike, and his children were of a similar age to Mike's, and he did not know how he would cope either. He could sense Mike's despair and distress and knew that the night is a very lonely time and a time where everything can seem so bleak. Mike was young and should have his whole life ahead of him and yet here he was with a devastating diagnosis.

Abdul said that he would not insult Mike's intelligence by saying everything would be alright – at this moment it must feel as if nothing would ever be right again. Mike clasped his arm and Abdul covered Mike's hand with his own and they sat looking at each other and talking about Mike's hopes and fears for some time. Abdul could not remember a time when it felt right to use touch as a means of support with another man of Mike's age, but it felt right now. Sometimes, with older men who were distressed, it had felt right, but men do not usually touch each other. However, he was, first and foremost, a nurse and he knew that many female nurses would have felt it was right to use therapeutic touch for such a situation. The fact that Abdul was male should not mean that Mike was denied this very personal form of human comfort and compassion. This was a time for such comfort and it felt as if it was an honour to share Mike's pain and be with him at his darkest time. He knew that he would remember this time with Mike for the rest of his life.

Discussion

Abdul was very busy that night, but this did not affect his ability to prioritise the fact that Mike needed to talk and was deeply distressed. He could sense his low mood from across the ward, and as soon as his other work demands eased a little and he knew that he had genuinely got time to spend with Mike, he treated Mike as his main priority. Abdul could see that Mike was awake and he could sense his agitation and restlessness. He then actively listened in an empathetic manner to his concerns and fears for the future. Once he was sure about the nature of Mike's fears, he gave him his attention and concentrated on what he was saying. He was assessing his psychological state, coping mechanisms and support networks, but this was all carried out with sensitivity and compassion. This fits in with the approach suggested by WONCA (2004) (World Organization of National Colleges, Academies and Academic Associations of General Practitioners/Family Physicians) of looking, listening and testing in relation to mental health status. Nurses might find this approach useful in ensuring that they respond appropriately to their clients' needs.

Abdul focused purely on the specific situation at the moment of communication (Rosengren 2000). He was aware of Mike's family situation, but most of all he was aware of his distress. In a Norwegian study, Hem and Heggen (2004) say that ignoring a patient's distress makes a patient feel lonely, and they suffer from a sense of not belonging. Mike was feeling very lonely at this point and Abdul's sensitive and empathetic approach was obviously highly valued by Mike. Attree (2001) says that good quality care is perceived by patients and relatives to be individualised, patient-focused and related to their needs. This needs to be provided humanistically through a caring relationship, acknowledging patients as individuals. Abdul exemplified all of these attributes in his approach to Mike.

Abdul's response focused more on what he did rather than what he said. It is easy to underestimate the importance of non-verbal skills. Abdul was calm and gave the impression that he had plenty of time and he was focused totally on Mike for the time he was with him. He sat down and, although he was aware of issues in relation to proximity, he felt that despite the fact that they were two men therapeutic touch was appropriate to ease Mike's distress.

A Welsh study on intimacy says that this includes some self-disclosure as well as trust, reciprocity and emotional closeness (Williams 2001). Therapeutic touch can convey caring, empathy and compassion, but touch involves an invasion of personal space, which can be threatening and intimidating or gentle and comforting. This depends on the situation, the individuals involved, the relationship and cultural norms. Abdul was very sensitive to all these factors and he felt that the use of touch was appropriate because it brought human comfort at a distressing time. Touch can be divided into 'instrumental' touch, which is deliberate physical contact necessary to perform a task, and 'affective or expressive' touch, which is relatively spontaneous and is not task orientated (Watson 1975 cited in Caris-Verhallen, Kerkstrar and Bensing 1999). This expressive touch was clearly valued by Mike on this occasion and was a clear example of responding appropriately to an individual person's needs.

THOUGHTS FOR YOUR PRACTICE

- How do you know that you understand the true message behind what your patients or clients are saying?
- Could you increase the extent to which your patients and clients are involved in decision making? If so, how?
- How can you prioritise times when you can focus on the individual needs of a patient, within a busy practice environment?
- How can you identify times when it is appropriate to use therapeutic touch in your interactions with patients and clients?
- Do you always feel that you provide as much comfort within your role as a nurse? If not, can you think of ways to strengthen this important part of your role?

Do we keep our focus on the patient while carrying out nursing tasks?

CASE STUDY 4.6

Akinyemi knew that he would die of AIDS and that death from AIDS was very common in his country. Despite this there was a lot of fear and a lack of understanding about the spread of the disease. At the moment, he was acutely unwell, but the times of remission were getting shorter and the healthcare in this remote part of Africa was very poor. There was not enough food or water, let alone medication, and any medication that was available was not of the expensive type that was needed to treat conditions such as his. He felt very vulnerable and frightened for both himself and his family.

Beatrice was nursing Akinyemi in the hut that they called a hospital. The tin roof made the heat unbearable during the long hours of sunshine. The temperature was getting higher all the time and it was still only 2:00pm. She was trying to keep Akinyemi as cool as possible to reduce his pyrexia. She kept a smile firmly on her face and maintained eye contact whenever she was close to him, but she had so many other patients to care for. She knew how important it was to provide reassurance, appear relaxed and be focused on each patient in the short time she spent with them.

Akinyemi felt reassured by Beatrice's presence and felt a sense of calm whenever she was near. She was always carrying out an aspect of care, but he still felt that she was emotionally involved with his situation and began to relax.

Discussion

Beatrice was very busy and had to focus on nursing tasks at all times, but she did not feel that that should mean she should not be focusing on Akinyemi as an individual whenever she was near him. There are different ways of carrying out nursing tasks – as just the task or as part of a holistic process. She made sure that she made eye contact as appropriate, and smiled and showed interest in Akinyemi as a person. McCabe (2004) differentiates between patient-centred communication and task-centred communication. When care is purely task orientated, the patient's needs can easily be ignored or compromised, which is detrimental to the relationship between nurse and patient.

Nurses should smile more to show patients they care about them and Beatrice was clearly doing this in her interactions with Akinyemi. As she was so busy, it would have been easy to say 'I'll be back in a minute' and not return. Patients then feel vulnerable, insecure and out of control, because they do not know if, or when, their needs will be met.

> Although technical ability and a general benevolent disposition towards people may mean one is a technically competent and not unkind nurse, the inspiration required to know what to say and when to say it, to capture the moment must, in my view, depend upon some degree of caring about the individual as a particular person. (De Raeve 1996, pp. 17–18)

De Raeve (2002) also differentiates between caring **for** a patient, which is task orientated, and caring **about** a patient, which involves an 'attitude of concern and commitment' (p. 159). Akinyemi would have been clear that Beatrice was not only caring for him, but also caring about him.

THOUGHTS FOR YOUR PRACTICE

- Do you always feel that you care about a patient as well as caring for them?
- How do you ensure that they feel cared about, as well as cared for?
- Are you sometimes unable to focus on more than the nursing tasks that need to be completed?
- If so, how can you start to change this?

SUMMARY – LINKS TO COMPASSION AND CARING

This chapter should have helped you to differentiate between listening, active listening and hearing what a person is actually saying. The importance of being able to allow adequate time to hear the patient's perspective as part of the assessment process cannot be overestimated. Listening to what is being said, and not said, can make the difference between poor practice and compassionate nursing. In busy practice environments, time can be very limited. However, there can be quieter times when nurses can focus on patients that they need to spend more time with. Often this precious time is used to catch up with paperwork, which, although important, can be less of a priority at that particular time.

There are genuine barriers to effective listening and you might want to spend some time thinking about how these barriers can be reduced in your practice area. Taking time to listen to patient narratives and the priorities people have are essential for person-centred nursing care.

Once someone has been listened to and heard, nurses need to respond appropriately to what is being said. This involves shared decision making and acting as an advocate, as appropriate. Sometimes the opportunity to listen and respond is a one-off opportunity that the nurse will never get again. This opportunity needs to be capitalised on in order for future care not to be compromised. Therapeutic touch can be part of such an 'appropriate response'; it has to be used carefully, but in many cases it is the most effective means of providing human comfort.

It is easy to focus on the nursing tasks to be carried out rather than the individuals themselves, in which case the patient is unlikely to feel cared for, let alone cared about. As Rungapadiachy (1999) says 'listening without responding is seen as hollow listening' (p. 221). Hollow listening does not in any way equate to caring or compassionate care.

REFERENCES

Attree M. Patients' and relatives' experiences and perspectives of 'good' and 'not so good' quality care. *J Adv Nurs.* 2001; **33**(4): 456–66.

Bordiak S. It is never acceptable to patronize clients. *Nurs Times.* 2008; **104**(9): 10.

Caris-Verhallen W, Kerkstrar A, Bensing J. Non-verbal behaviour in nurse-elderly patient communication. *J Adv Nurs.* 1999; **24**(4): 808–18.

De Raeve L. Caring intensively. In: Greaves D, Upton H, editors. *Philosophical Problems in Health Care.* Avebury: Aldershot; 1996: 9–22.

De Raeve L. Trust and trustworthiness in nurse-patient relationships. *Nursing Philosophy.* 2002; **3**(2): 152–62.

Egan G. *You and Me: the skills of communicating and relating to others.* Monterey, CA: Brooks/Cole; 1977.

Ewles L, Simnett I. *Promoting Health: a practical guide.* 5th ed. London: Balliere Tindall; 2003.

Harteveldt R. Holistic care is a major nursing achievement. *Nurs Times.* 2008; **104**(10): 12.

Hawkins J, Lindsay E. We listen but do we hear? The importance of patient stories. *Br J Community Nurs.* 2006; **11**(9): S6–14.

Hem M, Heggen K. Is compassion central to nursing practice? *Contemp Nurse.* 2004; **17**(1–2): 19–31.

Jonas-Simpson C, Mitchell G, Fisher A, *et al.* The experience of being listened to: a qualitative study of older adults in long-term care settings. *J Gerontol Nurs.* 2006; **32**(1): 46–54.

McCabe C. Nurse-patient communication: an exploration of patients' experiences. *J Clin Nurs.* 2004; **13**(1): 41–9.

Montori V, Gafni A, Charles C. A shared treatment decision-making approach between patients with chronic conditions and their clinicians: the case of diabetes. *Health Expect.* 2006; **9**(1): 25–36.

Rosengren K. *Communication: an introduction.* London: Sage Publications; 2000.

Rungapadiachy D. *Interpersonal Communication and Psychology for Healthcare Professionals.* Oxford: Butterworth Heinemann; 1999.

Stuart P, Knott D. Communication in end-of-life cardiac care 2: skills. *Nurs Times.* 2008; **104**(11): 26–7.

Vora E, Vora A. A contingency framework for listening to the dying. *Int Journal of Listening.* 2008; **22**: 59–72.

Williams A. A literature review on the concept of intimacy in nursing. *J Adv Nurs.* 2001; **33**(5): 660–7.

Wolvin A, Coakley C. *Listening.* 5th ed. Madison, WI: Brown and Benchmark Publisher; 1996.

WONCA Special Interest Group in Psychiatry and Neurology. *Culturally Sensitive Depression Guideline.* London: WONCA; 2004.

www.patientopinion.org.uk/opinion.aspx?opinionID=7838

CHAPTER 5

Diversity and cultural competence

Overview of the chapter

Key theme one – diversity
- Case study
- Discussion
- How do we identify individuals who are socially excluded?
- Case study
- Discussion
- Thoughts for your practice
- How can we ensure that our practice is as socially inclusive as possible?
- Case study
- Discussion
- Thoughts for your practice

Key theme two – cultural competence
- Case study
- Discussion
- How do we increase cultural awareness in nursing practice?
- Case study
- Discussion
- Thoughts for your practice
- Do we understand the importance of using cultural knowledge, skills and sensitivity in nursing practice?
- Case study
- Discussion
- Thoughts for your practice
- Summary – links to compassion and caring
- References

OVERVIEW OF THE CHAPTER

So far, all the chapters have focused on how compassion and caring centres on perceiving people as individuals with their own personal needs, rather than patients with problems or conditions. This chapter will focus on the very different ways that people perceive life and life choices, and how this impacts on individualised nursing care.

The importance of valuing difference in individuals and not stereotyping people into homogeneous groups is central to someone feeling that they are a person in their own right in a health service, which can feel institutionalised and impersonal. Diversity will therefore be the first major focus in this chapter.

For nurses to be able to provide an individualised approach to people in their care, they need to appreciate not only the diversity of their patients or clients, but also they need to become culturally competent in how they try to interpret differing needs and values. This means understanding that cultural norms can vary within seemingly homogeneous groups.

Therefore, this chapter will focus on diversity and cultural competence as key aspects of providing an individualised approach to nursing care. We hope that this will help you to further develop your thinking in relation to how you can provide optimal compassionate care in varying situations.

KEY THEME ONE – DIVERSITY

CASE STUDY 5.1

Libby feels misunderstood by lots of people. They don't understand the many problems she faces just trying to live her life and bring up her children. Her partner, Tony, is in prison again and she really thinks that he has an easier time of it than she does. After all, he doesn't have to bring up six children on his own. On his last brief spell in between prison stays she managed to get pregnant again, which is the last thing she needed, but he refuses to let her do anything to prevent future pregnancies. She really doesn't know what her GP will say. He wasn't very impressed when she got pregnant last time and Shannon is only three months old now. Her GP thinks she has got too much on her plate and she thinks that he is right.

She plucked up the courage to see her health visitor, Trudy, today and was pleasantly surprised by how it went. She had arranged to see Trudy before her appointment with the midwife, which was at the surgery. The appointment started badly, she was a bit late and had to take all six kids with her, which was never a good idea as it was difficult to keep them quiet in a strange environment with nothing to do. She felt that everyone else was looking down on her with their happy smiles and 'happy to be pregnant' looks and doting husbands, while she just felt desperate. She was happy for them, but it just wasn't the same for her.

Trudy actually seemed pleased to see her again, but was concerned by how tired she looked. She really seemed interested in how she was and how she was coping with everything. They had discussed the best way for Libby to have appointments with the midwife and Trudy seemed to understand the difficulties Libby had just going to appointments. Libby then felt more able to discuss this with the midwife who she had never met before.

Overall, Libby left the appointment feeling as if her needs were important to Trudy rather than feeling as if she was viewed as a problem, which is how she had previously felt on many occasions.

Discussion

Diversity can be seen as 'social variety across and within groups of people' (Thompson 2003, p. 10).

Society is made up of people of different:
➤ cultures
➤ races/nationalities
➤ abilities
➤ ages
➤ sexual identities
➤ religions/beliefs
➤ lifestyles.

All should have equality of opportunity for achieving their potential in relation to:
➤ health
➤ employment
➤ education
➤ housing
➤ civil rights
➤ self-actualisation.

Thompson discusses the importance of recognising and valuing the positive attributes of a group of people, as opposed to seeing diversity as a problem to be solved. He says that equal opportunities policies can focus too much on avoiding discrimination, under anti-discriminatory legislation, which is a defensive approach.

Baxter (2001) says 'managing diversity has a more positive message in relation to the overall organisational benefits of valuing and capitalising on the different backgrounds, characteristics and experiences of all employees' (p. 10). It is important that equal opportunities are not used in a managerial manner, in terms of doing the minimum to avoid legislative action, but to genuinely seek ways of increasing opportunities for those who have tradition- ally been disadvantaged.

Libby is definitely in a position of disadvantage in many different ways. She is trying to bring up six children, mainly on her own. Added to this, she is expecting another baby and cannot possibly be working and must exist on benefits, which puts her at an employment disadvantage. Her ethnic back- ground is not known; neither is her educational status, but she could be unable to read or write and be at an educational disadvantage. She is already at a health disadvantage, as are her children, because eating a nutritious diet is probably very difficult to afford on the money she has. She might also smoke, so this combined with everything else would also negatively impact on the health of her unborn baby. Her accommodation is bound to be cramped due to the size of her family and she is probably disadvantaged from a housing point of view. Her civil liberties are compromised due to her partner's views on contraception and she is definitely not able to self-actualise and fulfill her potential in life.

All of these factors might cause health professionals to act in a judgemental or patronising way towards her. However, she was treated with courtesy and respect by both professionals involved. They also made her feel important, valued and liked as an individual and she was consulted about her care needs. Too often a judgemental attitude is adopted by professionals when individuals do not attend for appointments or do not follow health advice, when no attempts have been made to understand the situation from the client's perspective. Therefore, it is not surprising that the relationship with a client or patient is set up to fail from the start. There might be no possible recovery from a relationship that starts off in a judgemental manner. In terms of diversity this is important. As Thompson (2003) says, the word diversity is becoming more popular because it is a positive term that 'emphasises the differences between individuals and across groups and the fact that such differences are best seen as assets to be valued and affirmed, rather than as problems to be solved' (p. 34).

The perception that 'difference' is a problem is the key component to individuals feeling undervalued. The 'asset approach' is advocated, where individuals are seen as an asset rather than a problem. Libby's situation is perceived as an asset because it allows the midwife and health visitor to meet her needs in a different way. However, in a pressurised health service it is understandable why her situation would not always be seen as an asset and Libby would then be blamed for not fitting in with a service that seems to work for most pregnant women. Meeting the needs of those whose needs are often highly complex, and who are often perceived as victims of the health inequalities divide, is essential for nurses and health visitors in order to address the public health agenda, in terms of the needs of populations as well as individuals.

How do we identify individuals who are socially excluded?

CASE STUDY 5.2

Goran could not remember a time when he had not been frightened. His country had been in a state of war for some years and he knew that his parents and grandparents had been frightened too, because there had always been a feeling of tension in the house whenever voices and sounds were heard from outside.

On that terrible night when they were woken by loud bangs and shouting and his parents had been dragged outside, he ran into his little sisters' room, grabbed the two terrified toddlers and had taken them to the hole in the wall behind the bed, which his parents had shown him. They knew better than to cry or make a sound; they had also grown up in this world of fear. He covered their ears and held them close as he heard the horrible sounds of gunfire nearby.

Goran had managed to walk at night with his sisters to the town 10 miles away, although it had taken several days, as they slept in hedges during the day. He found the home of his uncle who had somehow managed to get him sent to this strange country where he knew no one. He did not speak English, though he was trying to learn fast. He missed his family every day, but he knew that they were no longer alive and that he had to be strong for his sisters who relied on him. He was only nine years old and it felt as if the weight of the world was on his shoulders.

He was visited regularly by nurses who seemed to care and he was trying to study hard at school so that he could get a good job when he was old enough. He knew how lucky he was that they had managed to keep his family together. He felt so lonely, though, and his experiences and the fact that he spoke a different language made it difficult to talk to other children at school and he knew that they did not know what to make of him.

Discussion

Goran is clearly a member of a community who not only feel socially excluded, but also can be treated with a lack of understanding and criticism by the communities in which they now live. In some countries, asylum seekers have often received a lot of bad press in the media, as they are seen to be different from the indigenous community and a drain on the resources available to an area. There have been reports of some individuals who are seemingly seeking asylum, but who are trying to come to another country to have a better life-style, rather than escape fear and tyranny in their home country. Individuals in their new country of residence then feel resentful and angry that they should be allowed to do this, and genuine asylum seekers can feel much excluded by their new community.

Goran (and his sisters) are in the looked-after system, and are clearly disadvantaged in this way too. He is an unaccompanied minor who needs to be cared for until he is old enough to be independent. Other young men, older than Goran, are also disadvantaged because any benefits they may be receiving may be very minimal and eating healthily and finding work can be impossible for them. Again this can lead to a judgemental approach by others. There are many potential levels of disadvantage for Goran and his sisters. Educationally, he is trying to learn in another country, where he does not speak the language. Socially, he does not feel as if he fits in with his peers at school, or with others outside his school environment. He cannot live the carefree life of his contemporaries, because he has his sisters to worry about and he is not socially and culturally acclimatised to his new world. Potentially, he could end up living in poverty and be dependent on benefits in the future if he did not have a strong personal work ethic. Of course he is also bereaved in terms of the loss of members of his close family, which leaves him extremely emotionally vulnerable and socially isolated.

Goran is a classic example of someone who is socially excluded. Silver (2007) defines social exclusion as '. . . a multi-dimensional process of progressive social rupture, detaching groups and individuals from social relations and institutions and preventing them from full participation in the normal, normatively prescribed activities of the society in which they live' (p. 15). He goes on to say 'whatever the content and criteria of social membership, socially excluded groups and individuals lack capacity or access to social opportunity' (p. 15). The point that Silver is making is that a community, or society, prescribes their own norms and values, plus who is considered to fit in with those norms and values, and who does not. In many cases, there is no accepted, or perhaps verbalised, definition of who should, or should not, live in that community. However, the implicit view is that certain people should be included and others would remain on the outside. In many cases, this assumption is not related to a specific individual, but people are prejudged merely because they do not fit in with the locally prescribed definition of what is considered to be an acceptable member of the community. Therefore, they do lack access to opportunities for social engagement.This situation can become more pronounced as time goes by and future individuals can be excluded before they even move into an area. There is no commitment in these situations to trying to resolve these issues, or trying to get to know individuals and break down barriers that marginalise people and groups within society.

In the UK, the Salvation Army (2008) discuss the fact that social exclusion relates to the alienation or disenfranchisement of certain people within a society. This can be related to many different, potentially disadvantaged individuals and populations and can also be influenced by people's social class, living standards and educational status, such as:

➤ people with a disability;
➤ minority men and women of all races;
➤ older people;
➤ young people;
➤ teenage parents;
➤ those who are vulnerably housed;
➤ those who are socially isolated;
➤ those who are rurally isolated;
➤ prisoners and ex-offenders;
➤ working women;
➤ people with learning needs;
➤ Black and minority ethnic groups;
➤ looked-after children;
➤ asylum seekers;
➤ those who cannot read or write;
➤ travelling families;

➤ substance misusers;
➤ people with mental health needs;
➤ those for whom English is not their first language.

This list is not meant to be exhaustive, or, in fact, imply that all people in these situations are disadvantaged, but merely that we should all be looking for people who may be excluded within our society. For example, it would be easy for a nurse working in a neonatal unit to judge a mother, who is a lone parent, for not visiting her newborn baby as frequently as other parents. This would not be taking into account the needs of her other children, the fact that she is living in a rurally isolated area with no public transport, or the expense of getting to the hospital and the care of her other children. We can plan different strategies to meet the differing needs of our patients and clients, and provide resources that are more responsive to those different needs.

The wide variation in health opportunity and health status has been discussed for some years, along with the social determinants that underlie these. The World Health Organization (WHO) (2008) is committed to closing this gap within and between countries.

> Access to and utilisation of healthcare is vital to good and equitable health. The healthcare system is itself a social determinant of health, influenced by and influencing the effect of other social determinants. Gender, education, occupation, income, ethnicity, and place of residence are all closely linked to people's access to, experiences of, and benefits from healthcare. (WHO 2008, p. 16)

They point out how wide these variations can be and say that 'social justice is a matter of life and death'. It affects the way people live, the consequent chance of illness, and their risk of premature death. We watch in wonder as life expectancy and good health continue to increase in parts of the world and in alarm as they fail to improve in others. A girl born today can expect to live for more than 80 years if she is born in some countries – but less than 45 years if she is born in others. Even within countries there are dramatic differences in health that are closely linked with degrees of social disadvantage. Differences of this magnitude, within and between countries, simply should never happen. These inequities in health, avoidable health inequalities, arise because of the circumstances in which people grow, live, work, and age, and the systems put in place to deal with illness (WHO 2008).

As far back at 1999, a Department of Health (DOH) document in the UK stated that: 'Health inequality is widespread. The most disadvantaged have suffered most from ill health' (DOH 1999). More recently in the UK, Shaw, Davey Smith and Dorling (2005) commented that the poorest 10% in society received 3% of the nation's total income, while the richest 10% received more than 25%. This is clearly very iniquitous and leaves individuals and groups within society at a severe disadvantage. The UK Human Rights Act (Home Office 1998) said that everyone had the right not to be discriminated against on the grounds of race or gender or in the enjoyment of their conventional rights.

Black (1994, cited in Robinson and Elkan 1996) states the importance of understanding how certain people can be disadvantaged and points out that some people can be doubly or triply disadvantaged. Goran, for example, is disadvantaged by his traumatic recent life, his inability to speak the language of the country where he is living, his ethnicity being different from those around of them, his lack of family and his bereavement. Others could be disadvantaged by education, poverty, illness, disability and cultural isolation.

In order to try to counteract the health inequalities that there are, nurses need to understand the principles of vertical and horizontal equity. Gerrish and Papadopoulos (1999) say that **horizontal equity** is equal treatment to equals, whereas **vertical equity** is unequal but appropriate treatment to those with unequal needs. Therefore, any service or benefit that is offered to everyone, regardless of need, is not taking into account the fact that some people could afford to pay for this service, while others cannot. Vertical equity tries to reduce the effect of inequality by offering more services to those most in need. Gerrish and Papadopoulos (1999) also say that 'a failure to recognise the disadvantaged position of minority and ethnic communities is likely to result in an inappropriate focus on the principles of horizontal equity to the neglect of addressing vertical equity' (p. 1454).

This discussion should have helped you to understand in greater depth the factors that can make some people more vulnerable to ill health and premature death and how people can be excluded from society in a way that further increases their disadvantage in life. As nurses, we need to concentrate on ways to seek out those at risk of social exclusion and health disadvantage and find more ways of meeting the needs of our diverse communities. The next section will discuss some ways of minimising health disadvantage in nursing practice.

THOUGHTS FOR YOUR PRACTICE

- How do you think that you can increase the opportunities to develop your practice in a way that meets the needs of the full potential diversity of your client group?
- How can your encourage this approach within your practice team?
- How can you increase your ability to see individuals who do not fit with your own social norms as an asset rather than a problem?
- What areas of potential social exclusion have you experienced in individuals and families that you have nursed?
- How has this disadvantage manifested itself to you?
- Can you identify individuals and groups who are more disadvantaged in relation to health?
- Can you think about ways in which the principles of vertical equity could be used to enhance the life and health chances of these individuals and groups?

How can we ensure that our practice is as socially inclusive as possible?

CASE STUDY 5.3

Doris had been greatly shocked by her emergency admission to hospital. She thought that she had indigestion and a bit of neck pain and was thinking of having a bit of a lie down when her granddaughter, Amy, popped in to see her on the way back from school. Amy had been full of her school day. She had been to see round the hospital emergency department and the half-day session had also taught her how to help people who were suffering from sudden onset illnesses, such as an epileptic fit, a stroke and a heart attack. Doris liked to hear Amy talk about her day and when she was listening to her talking about the symptoms of a heart attack she jokingly said that those symptoms must be very common because she had had some of those all afternoon.

To her surprise Amy was suddenly in full action, phoning the local doctor's surgery and telling them about her gran's symptoms. The next thing she knew an ambulance had arrived and two calm and friendly paramedics were plugging her up to a monitor and taking her to hospital.

She had spent a few days in hospital and had been told that she had definitely had a heart attack and that she was very lucky that her granddaughter had recognised the fact that she was ill and had sought help so fast.

Now she was just about to be discharged from hospital and the nurse on the cardiac ward, who had introduced herself as Lucy, was trying to discuss things that would help her health in the future. The problem was that she was describing things that would not be possible for her at all. Although Lucy had obviously realised that Doris was on a pension and short of money, she did not appear to understand the practical problems involved for Doris to follow her advice.

Doris lived in a flat on the 12th floor and the lift did not work most of the time. When it did, it smelt of urine and you never really knew who was around and whether it was safe or not. The reality of buying fresh fruit and vegetables on a regular basis was really not a possibility for Doris. Those sorts of food had to be bought frequently, and could be expensive. The local shop stocked a bit of fruit, but it was usually not in the best condition, did not last long and was expensive. Also, it was very heavy to carry back to her flat – whether the lift was working or not. She could not ask her busy daughter to shop for her that often. She found herself drifting away from the conversation and heard herself mumbling agreement. Lucy went away, obviously pleased that she had given Doris the information she needed.

Discussion

Lucy had the best of intentions in trying to give Doris pre-discharge information. However, it was clear that she was not actually having a conversation with Doris; she was just giving her general health advice that would be given to anybody following a myocardial infarction. It would not have been possible for Lucy to have known anything about Doris's home situation unless she had asked her. It can be much easier in a busy ward situation to go through the motions and give health advice or health education, without really understanding what will work with the person's life and lifestyle. Unfortunately, the next step on from this is to blame the individual when something goes wrong, because they have not followed health advice.

In the UK, inequalities in health are evident in many different health conditions. For example in relation to coronary heart disease, the National Service Framework for Coronary Heart Disease (DOH 2000) highlights the following:

> More than 110 000 people die of heart problems in England every year.
> But the effects of heart disease are unequal: among unskilled men the
> death rate is almost three times higher than it is among professionals.
> These differences have more than doubled in the past 20 years. Heart
> disease is much more common in deprived areas, yet treatment and care
> is often better in more prosperous areas. This 'postcode' lottery of care is
> unacceptable (p. 2).
> Angina, heart attack and stroke are all more common among those in
> manual classes (p. 6).
> There are also ethnic variations for people born in the Indian
> subcontinent; the death rate for heart disease is 38% higher for men and
> 43% higher for women than rates for the country as a whole (p. 6).

If these inequalities are to be minimised, then advice has to be appropriate
to people who have less money, who live in deprived areas or who are unable
to eat foods that have traditionally been eaten by others of their ethnic group
for generations. If Lucy had asked Doris what she normally ate, where she
normally shopped, what sort of environment she lived in and who could help
her to buy food at times, they might have been able to jointly come up with
some solutions to the difficulties that Doris thought were insurmountable.
However, Lucy's approach did not allow for this discussion to take place.

While Doris is an example of a person experiencing inequalities in relation to heart disease, as nurses we must be aware that similar inequalities can
be replicated with individuals with other health issues. For example, people
with mental health issues are more likely to be unemployed, living in poverty,
vulnerably housed, offenders or ex-offenders, victims of domestic abuse or
substance misusers. In addition, there are patterns to people who are more
likely to suffer from mental health problems: they are often men from the Afro
Carribean or women with a background from the Indian subcontinent (DOH
1999). These women are not only at greater risk, but they are disadvantaged
by the fact that mental health issues are very much stigmatised within this
cultural group. Diagnosis is more difficult and access to assessment, treatment and care is inhibited by a lack of understanding of the manifestations
of depression in this ethnic group and a stigmatisation within the community
in which they live. Without an understanding of these issues this disadvantage
will continue within this ethnic community.

Race is a major factor in health generally. Ali and Atkin (2004) raise concerns about healthcare services not necessarily being available to meet the
needs of different ethnic groups. They make the point that offering the same

service for all equates to an equal service for all (horizontal equity) and often problems will arise due to genuine ignorance, a deliberate failure to engage with difference or being so overwhelmed by the difficulties in providing care to a multi-ethnic population that offering a generic service is the easiest option. There can be higher rates of coronary heart disease and diabetes in these communities (Robotham and Sheldrake 2000), so those working to reduce levels of ill health in relation to these health conditions need to work towards providing a service to meet the needs of all people in the community in which they work.

When two potentially disadvantaging factors are combined, this can doubly impact on an individual's health. For example, if an older person is from a different ethnic background to that which is most common in that country or that geographical area, that person might experience more discrimination in accessing services. If that person also suffers from mental health problems it adds a triple disadvantage. The UK National Service Framework for Older People (DOH 2001) says that such people need more accessible and more appropriate mental health services. Some of the difficulties are that

➤ assessment must have a cultural bias to overcome difficulties in identifying needs;
➤ there can be assumptions made about the willingness and capability of families to act as primary carers;
➤ the information might not be accessible if not translated into their language but it cannot be assumed that everybody can read the language that they speak;
➤ the services might not be readily accessible or fully appropriate;
➤ where this has happened there may be distrust of agencies by some Black and minority ethnic communities.

Another example of a double health disadvantage can be that of being a woman who has a mental health problem. Mental health problems present in unique ways and individuals can be at greater risk, or be protected by, their gender. Nurses need to be aware of how mental health and gender interrelate. For example, women can have better social networks than men and can have positive experiences in relation to motherhood and family links. However, they can also have negative life experiences that contribute to their mental health problems, such as:

➤ rape, sexual abuse, domestic violence;
➤ hormonal influences;
➤ negative life events;

➤ social isolation;
➤ poverty due to childcare responsibilities that reduce work opportunities.

A UK paper on women and mental health (DOH 2002) states that women who are particularly at risk of mental health problems are
➤ women who are mothers or carers;
➤ older women;
➤ women from Black and minority groups;
➤ lesbian and bisexual women;
➤ transsexual women;
➤ women involved in prostitution;
➤ women offenders;
➤ women with learning disabilities;
➤ women who misuse alcohol or drugs.

However, when considering the needs of women, it is also important to emphasise the needs of men. Men can be very disadvantaged when accessing healthcare. They tend to be much less familiar with healthcare services because women are often more likely to access them in their roles as child bearer or caregiver. Therefore, women may feel more comfortable in the healthcare environment. Men often approach a healthcare professional because they have been advised to do so by their partner, and often use this as a reason for attending a clinic. They feel that it is not 'manly' to admit to health problems and tend to ignore symptoms and make excuses for not accessing help. Galdas, Cheater and Marshall (2005) say that 'there is a growing trend in the literature indicating that "male socialisation" may have an adverse effect on men's health, with, in particular, a reluctance to seek help when they experience illness' (p. 621). It is very important for nurses to realise the reluctance with which men approach healthcare services and adapt their approach to take this into account. An informal but professional approach, which reassures a man that he is not wasting anybody's time and that he was right to seek help, can encourage him to do so on future occasions.

In addition, rather as young people need to have an individualised approach to how nurses communicate with them, so do older people. Older people can feel discriminated against when it comes to the use of healthcare resources. It is easy for them to feel that others see it as a waste to spend precious healthcare time and resources on someone of their advanced years.

NHS services will be provided, regardless of age, on the basis of clinical need alone. Social care agencies will not use age in their eligibility criteria or policies, to restrict access to available services. Decisions about treatment and care should be made on the basis of each individual's health needs not their age. Even very complex treatment, used appropriately, can benefit older people and should not be denied them solely on the basis of age. (UK National Service Framework for Older People, DOH 2001, p. 6)

It is important for nurses to realise that people with disabilities, or those suffering from significant long-term conditions, can be very socially excluded and disadvantaged. As the UK National Service Framework for Long Term Conditions (DOH 2005) says, 'the social model of disability recognises that social and environmental barriers limit opportunities for disabled people to take part in society on an equal basis with other people' (p. 74).

There are many people with whom we come into contact within our nursing practice who are potentially disadvantaged and socially excluded. As nurses, it is our role to ensure that this disadvantage and exclusion is minimised as far as possible. Understanding diversity, in all its manifestations, is essential to providing socially inclusive care, and key to this is increasing our level of cultural competence in order to enhance our compassionate nursing care.

THOUGHTS FOR YOUR PRACTICE

- How can you increase your level of awareness, sensitivity and responsiveness to the differing needs in your patient or client group?
- Can you think of ways to be proactive in improving the nursing practice where you work to reduce the possibility of social exclusion?
- Reflect on your practice in relation to the different client groups highlighted in this section.
- Think of a specific patient from one of these client groups.
- How did you ensure that you identified their potential health inequalities?
- What action did you take to minimise these inequalities?
- Can you think of any other client groups who need to have a more socially inclusive approach to their care in your practice area?
- How do you intend to ensure that your practice, and that of others, is as socially inclusive as possible?

KEY THEME TWO – CULTURAL COMPETENCE

CASE STUDY 5.4

Several times in the past, Suri had been admitted to the same ward with ulcerative colitis, but on admission this time the nurse seemed to be really interested in finding out what was important to her, and what her needs would be while she was on the ward. Previously, Suri had had reservations about male nurses because she had been concerned about how she would feel about discussing intimate things concerning her body with a man. However, this nurse, who had introduced himself as Dave, seemed to be really interested in her needs and preferences. In the past, nurses on the ward had tried to hide their lack of knowledge of Suri's cultural background by making sweeping statements about what they assumed Suri might want, based on other women from the same ethnic background who had been patients there before. Didn't they know that her views were her own, and not totally determined by her ethnic background? They never seemed relaxed with Suri and appeared to be constantly worried about saying the wrong thing and this made Suri feel on edge too.

In comparison, Dave started off by saying that he was recently qualified and had not met many women of her ethnic background and would like to make sure that Suri's stay in the ward went as she would want it to. He offered to change with a female colleague if she was not comfortable with having a male nurse. He also said that he would welcome the opportunity to gain some insight into how her cultural background influenced her choices. He seemed comfortable and open with her, and she felt relaxed from the start.

Discussion

Campinha-Bacote (2002) states that cultural competence is a process and not an event and Dave is recognising this by showing that he has some cultural **awareness**, but would like to develop his cultural **knowledge** and **skill** further by capitalising on his cultural **encounters**. Through this, he is demonstrating a **desire** to be more culturally competent. These are the five constructs of cultural competence according to Campinha-Bacote (1999), and it is important to understand that there are more variations within ethnic groups than across them. Problems can arise when people do not understand this and make sweeping assumptions based on ethnic group alone. Dave is clearly demonstrating to Suri that he has a strong motivation to provide ethnically sensitive and individualised care, and that he is entering a professional partnership with her that is based on mutual respect and increased knowledge on both sides.

As already indicated, Campinha-Bacote's (1999) model contains five constructs:

1 **Cultural awareness** – awareness and sensitivity to the values, beliefs and problem solving strategies of clients' cultures.
2 **Cultural knowledge** – seeking and gaining knowledge of various world views of different cultures.
3 **Cultural skill** – the ability to collect relevant cultural data regarding a client's health history and presenting problems as well as carrying out an appropriate culturally specific assessment.
4 **Cultural encounters** – the process that encourages healthcare providers to engage directly in cross cultural interactions with people from different cultures.
5 **Cultural desire** – the motivation of healthcare providers to 'want to' engage in the process of cultural competence. This includes a genuine desire and motivation to work with different people and having a genuine interest in the individual.

Papadopoulos, Tilki and Taylor (1998) introduce a further construct of **cultural sensitivity**. This includes a person's ability to be empathetic, appropriate and accepting, using good interpersonal communication skills, which help to generate trust and respect. Chen and Starosta (2000) devised a toolkit to measure cultural sensitivity, which covers six elements:

➤ self-esteem
➤ self-monitoring
➤ open-mindedness
➤ empathy
➤ interaction involvement
➤ no judgement.

Dave was clearly demonstrating **cultural sensitivity** through his high level of interpersonal skills, which were evident in his empathy, self-knowledge and awareness, and his non-judgemental attitude in perceiving Suri as an individual in her own right. Therefore, he was demonstrating cultural competence, which Husain (2005) perceives as the overlap area between cultural knowledge, awareness and sensitivity.

It is easy to make assumptions and generalise care when this is not the intention (Hilgenberg and Schlickau 2002). Dave is not falling into this trap and is aware of the gaps in his knowledge. As a newly qualified practitioner, it is perhaps easier for him to be aware of his total lack of knowledge of cultural behaviour and needs. If he had had contact with many women from Suri's ethnic group, he might have made unconscious assumptions about her cultural needs. Cultural awareness is essential to nurses delivering culturally sensitive care. For example, just because there might be a large community from a particular ethnic background living locally, it could be wrongly assumed that all nurses working with that community would be aware of how such cultural norms might affect their planning of care. In addition, if a woman from a different ethnic background is living in an area where she is culturally isolated, her care might be compromised by a lack of knowledge of cultural variations. These are essential points in caring for people in a culturally sensitive manner.

> Clients often view nursing care negatively when the care fails to fit with their life ways, needs, and expectations. Misunderstandings, or different interpretations of the same phenomena as a result of the cultural differences, can lead to a lack of trust and respect between nurses and their clients. (Leininger 1995, cited in Kim-Godwin, Clarke and Barton 2001, p. 919)

Dave and Suri are of different ethnic backgrounds and, therefore, communication between them is intercultural (Jandt 2001). Dave is aware of this and of the fact that intercultural communication involves communication between people of diverse cultures, involving different norms and values.

Jandt (2001) states that stereotyping and prejudice can impede the communication that takes place. He defines stereotyping as 'negative or positive judgements made about individuals based on any observable or believed group membership' (p. 45). This point about positive stereotyping also being harmful is a sensitive issue, as many people believe that positive stereotyping is not a problem. For example, it is often assumed that people of Afro-Caribbean descent dance better than their Caucasian counterparts. However, this positive stereotyping allows individuals to be perceived as merely members of a group and not as individuals. There can be an element of fear or prejudice once someone's religious or ethnic allegiance is visible. For example, the religious allegiance of an individual who is Jewish, or someone of African origin who is also a Muslim, might not be as clearly evident as an Orthodox Jew or someone whose Muslim beliefs are clearly identified by their dress. Therefore, the more visible someone's allegiance to a group actually is, the more likely it is that this could lead to prejudice. Prejudice, according to Jandt (2001), is an 'irrational suspicion or hatred of a particular group, race, religion or orientation. Persons within the group are viewed not in terms of their individual merit, but according to the superficial characteristics that make them part of the group' (p. 45).

Thompson (2001) says 'there is no middle ground: intervention either adds to oppression (or at least condones it) or goes some small way towards easing or breaking such oppression' (p. 11). He goes on to say that 'in short, practice which does not take account of oppression and discrimination cannot be seen as good practice, no matter how high its standards may be in other respects'(p. 11). For example, a nurse who is caring for a person with a disability might provide excellent care within the hospital environment. However, they might not plan the discharge from hospital as effectively as they could because they are unaware of the difficulties that the individual faces at home on a day-to-day basis.

If Dave had not taken into account how individuals, ethnic groups and communities are marginalised within society and how their life chances and choices are limited by the way that the world perceives them, or by their financial or social status, then it would not have been possible to deliver client- or patient-focused care. Nurses can find themselves in the position of giving advice that is impractical or impossible for the patients in their care. This could lead to potential judgemental attitudes and behaviour when individuals are not able to follow advice. Dave tried to develop cultural knowledge about Suri's needs in order to deliver optimal care and to be able to work in partnership to meet her future health needs.

This scenario raises important issues about cultural competence and the importance of not stereotyping people from the same ethnic background as this can lead to non-individualised care and inaccurate assumptions about health needs and the nursing care required. The next section will focus on the importance of cultural awareness, and cultural knowledge and skills in delivering culturally competent care.

How do we increase cultural awareness in nursing practice?

CASE STUDY 5.5

Bill is not someone who uses healthcare services very much and he is only going to the health centre for immunisation advice before he goes on a trip to Brazil. He has made an appointment to see Ann, the practice nurse. He is only in his early forties but at the moment he feels a lot older. Generally, he feels well and is trying to look forward to his holiday; he is aware that he might need some vaccinations. A month ago his wife, Maureen, suddenly told him that she did not love him any more and wanted to be on her own. He knew that he had been neglecting her a bit because he was so busy at work, but he thought that she understood how important it was for both of them that he worked long hours just now. He had just set up his own business, which should have given them both a good lifestyle, but his heart was not in it now. He had heard from neighbours that she was not on her own and he did not know how long the affair had been going on while they were still together. He still loved her very much and felt very emotionally vulnerable and just hoped that this holiday might help him to feel more positive about his life. He was finding it very difficult to cope with life at the moment.

Ann, the practice nurse, greets Bill with a smile. She knows him well as he visits her for his asthma management. She asks him why he is visiting her today and is shocked at how demoralised and subdued he looks – not his usual cheerful self at all. His asthma is generally fairly well controlled, but he smokes 20 cigarettes a day and this has been having a negative impact on his general health. However, her concern today is in finding out how she can help him as he is obviously very unhappy. He tells Ann about his holiday plans and then starts to break down when he tells her about his wife. Ann feels very concerned about Bill's obvious distress and wants to focus not only on giving him the vaccinations he needs, but also on assessing his emotional state. They are the priorities today, not his asthma, and certainly not his smoking.

Discussion

Ann is very aware that Bill has his own individuality and cultural identity. As Cortis (2003) says, cultural identity is based on a person's beliefs and values as well as their sense of self-worth and belonging. Bill's sense of self-worth and belonging had been severely damaged by recent events and Ann is concerned about this. Bill's cultural identity is made up by the fact that he is a heterosexual Caucasian man in his early forties. He is also a strong believer in marriage, and he perceives himself to be a married man and, therefore, his beliefs, personal philosophy, role and relationships within society have been changed radically. He feels that his whole identity has been shaken. From Ann's perspective, she can see all those things in Bill, but also, from a nursing perspective, she sees him as a generally fit and well man who has asthma and smokes.

Ann's understanding of Bill's cultural identity is essential to her being able to be culturally aware in her discussions with him. She has some awareness of his values, beliefs and problem-solving strategies, which are important components of cultural awareness. Therefore, her focus today is not on his smoking, but on his emotional well-being and vulnerability.

Smoking cessation advice can be ineffective and poorly delivered, and smokers need to be seen as a cultural group with their own identity. Therefore, a culturally competent approach needs to be taken to ensure that the needs of people who smoke are met in an individual and non-judgemental manner in order for them to feel empowered to bring about a major life change. This would not have happened if Ann did not appreciate the inappropriateness of even mentioning smoking at today's visit. This would have been insensitive and ineffectual when he was feeling so vulnerable, and could potentially have delayed or prevented him feeling motivated to stop smoking in the future. A more personalised approach to smoking cessation can enhance the effectiveness of advice and hopefully lead to a more positive outcome in some cases. Nurses who may be non-smokers themselves need to have some awareness of the challenges and judgemental attitudes that smokers can face on a day-to-day basis. Otherwise a smoker's experience of health services can feel very negative. This can affect their life choices, which can, in turn, affect their capacity to maximise their health potential.

'Culture involves an integrated pattern of human behaviour that includes thoughts, communications, actions, customs, beliefs, values . . . [of a] social nature' (Chambers and Alexis 2004, p. 1357). In this case, Bill's culture would include the fact that he is a smoker, which gives him a different cultural identity from non-smokers. It is important to recognise this cultural identity in order to meet his health needs. When this is acknowledged, it is then possible to take a personalised approach to ensure that his unique needs are met as an individual. In order for Ann to start to address Bill's health needs, she needs to become competent at understanding the health needs associated with the group identity of people who smoke and then more specifically Bill's individual culture.

Cultural competence involves 'honouring and respecting a variety of beliefs, interpersonal styles, attitudes and behaviours' (Alexis and Chambers 2003, p. 29, Part 2). Although cultural competence is usually viewed particularly in relation to race and cultural identity, it is possible to see how a cultural identity could exist among people who smoke.

Smokers can feel very marginalised by society as the places where smoking is acceptable becomes ever smaller. In addition, healthcare professionals often focus on smoking cessation to the exclusion of other health needs, which might be more important from the client's perspective. Therefore, it is essential that healthcare professionals carry out a full assessment to determine what the client's health needs are at that stage and what the client hopes to gain from the consultation.

At every appointment, each client has their own particular agenda for what they hope to gain from the consultation. In this case, Bill's **expressed** needs are in relation to his travel vaccines, although he has underlying unexpressed and **felt** needs in relation to his emotional status. The professional perspective is that Ann has **normative** and **comparative** needs to discuss Bill's smoking and encourage him in smoking cessation (Bradshaw 1972). These differing perceptions of need can be a real hindrance in relationships and discussions between clients and nurses. Focusing on the professional agenda, to the detriment of the client's agenda, can negatively impact the outcome of a conversation.

Ann is concerned by Bill's change in demeanour and wants to try to find out the reason for this as part of the assessment process. Not only does she want to identify what vaccinations he might need, but also what other travel advice might be helpful. The fact that he is a smoker is clearly identified on his medical records on the computer screen and she is aware of the national guidelines that recommend that smoking is discussed at every consultation. Therefore, it would be tempting to address this normative agenda, to the detriment of assessing his mental health status. Bill knows that smoking is bad for him, and reminding him of this, and focusing on his smoking, might stop him from disclosing the more immediate and sensitive issues that are having more of an impact on his health at the moment.

Therefore, Ann starts by asking how he is feeling and says that she has noticed that he appears sad and withdrawn. Bill tells her about his marital problems and how he is not sleeping and finding it difficult to concentrate at work. He booked this holiday on impulse because he was aware that he needed something positive to look forward to. Ann gives him the opportunity to explore his feelings and express his regret about how the situation has deteriorated and how it is affecting him. She gives appropriate advice concerning the vaccinations required for Brazil, bearing in mind any possible contraindications in terms of his health status.

Ann does not always give smoking advice at every consultation because she feels that frequent attenders do not always respond well to this discussion at every visit and it can be counterproductive. She tries to discuss smoking in a manner that is appropriate to each consultation, individual and circumstance, rather than raising the topic every time. She is aware of the difficulties that individuals have when giving up smoking and that smokers develop their own culture by virtue of the fact that they are smokers.

Today, Ann is aware that Bill's state of mind might mean that giving up smoking is impossible for him at this time, although she knows that ideally he wants to try when he feels that the timing is right for him. She has been trying to empower him to feel that this could be a reality for him. However, she does feel that it would be appropriate to discuss how Bill is thinking of managing the long flight without smoking. Bill had not thought about this yet, but appreciated that this would be a problem for him. He then suggested that this would in fact be an ideal time to try to stop smoking as he would be in a different environment and away from everyday stresses and that, due to the long flights, he would be unable to smoke. Bill and Ann then started to have a concordant discussion about nicotine replacement therapy. Because this is now his decision, the conversation is much more positive, and his emotional needs have not been ignored.

Having discussed the importance of understanding cultural identity and being culturally aware, it is possible to see how nurses can further develop these constructs within their practice. However, they may also need to increase their cultural knowledge and skills, which will be discussed in the next section.

THOUGHTS FOR YOUR PRACTICE

- Have you ever thought about whether you are **culturally competent** in your practice?
- Think about ways in which you could increase your own **cultural sensitivity**, and that of others.
- How can you increase the level of **cultural desire** in colleagues and students who are less aware of these issues?
- How can you increase the opportunities for **cultural encounters** for yourself and students?
- If so, how do you ensure that you understand the **cultural identities** of different people in your care?
- If you have not had the opportunity to explore cultural competence in relation to your current practice, how would you try to increase this perspective in yourself and colleagues?
- Try to think about the cultural identities of two people that you

have nursed recently, one of whom might not have had a clearly recognisable cultural identity.

- What could you have done to enhance their experiences of their nursing care?
- How could you increase your cultural awareness of the values, beliefs and problem-solving strategies of people in your care?

Do we understand the importance of using cultural knowledge, skills and sensitivity in nursing practice?

CASE STUDY 5.6

Paul knew that he did not have much time left and yet there was a lot he felt he needed to do. It was not so much that he was frightened of death itself, but he was worried about the unresolved emotional issues that he would leave behind. His relationship with Rick was the best thing that had ever happened to him and he could not understand why, after all this time, his parents could not accept this. Rick had suggested that they celebrate their 20th anniversary together in Venice last year and the memories of that time were so important to him, yet his parents would not even look at his photographs. Rick had never been to Paul's parents' home. It had been made very clear that he would never be welcome and they never came to visit Paul in his home. In contrast, Rick's parents behaved more like they were his parents too. They celebrated their son's happiness and welcomed any contact with Paul.

Now he had been admitted to the hospice, on his own request. Rick had cared for him so lovingly, but he was exhausted and frightened about facing the loss of Paul on his own. He needed more support and the hospice certainly gave them both that. One nurse, Sue, had been particularly supportive about the issues they faced in bringing Paul's loved ones together.

At the moment Paul could hear his parents shouting outside the room where he and Rick and Rick's parents were. Paul felt embarrassed and sad that Rick was being rejected. He could hear his parents say that they were Paul's next of kin and had a right to say who should be with him when he was so ill. He could hear Sue asking in a calm voice what they were most worried about. He heard his mother saying that she was worried about not being with Paul as he became more ill, because

Rick was there so much of the time. Sue then asked what they thought would bring Paul most peace. There was silence and no response. She quietly said, 'Wouldn't he want you all to be free to visit him, together and individually and to feel that Rick was accepted by the parents that he also loved so much?' Again silence. Sue went on to say how obvious it was that Paul and Rick loved each other very much and that Rick was devastated by the loss he faced. She was sure that Paul would feel comforted to know that his parents would be there to help Rick to cope with this immense lost that she knew that they would all feel. Although the silence continued, Paul saw the door open and his parents walked in. He had never seen his father cry before, but his mother kissed Rick on the cheek and his father shook his hand without making eye contact. It was a start.

Discussion

Sue was clearly using all her advanced communication skills, tact, diplomacy, negotiating and problem-solving skills in this very difficult situation. If she had not perceived Paul and Rick's **cultural identity** as both male and as a loving homosexual couple, she would not have understood their norms and beliefs and the problems they might face in being accepted by some parts of society – in this case Paul's parents. She was therefore **culturally aware** and used her **cultural knowledge** and **cultural sensitivity** to negotiate and problem solve at a high level.

Campinha-Bacote (2002) stresses the importance of obtaining **cultural knowledge** about the client's values and beliefs in order to understand their perspective on life, which guides their 'thinking, doing and being' (p. 182).

> In obtaining cultural knowledge, it is critical to remember that no individual is a stereotype of one's own culture of origin, but rather a unique blend of the diversity found within each culture, a unique accumulation of life experiences, and the process of acculturation to other cultures. Therefore, the healthcare provider must develop the ability to conduct a cultural assessment with each client. (Campinha-Bacote 2002, p. 182)

Paul and Rick have their own unique relationship, perspectives and views on life, which include the importance of being accepted by their families. Papadopoulos and Lees (2002) stress the importance of understanding similarities and differences within a cultural group, but also not making the assumption that 'there are essential cultural differences between people which always override other aspects of their being' (p. 261). They make the point that this 'can lead to stereotyping, prejudice and discrimination' (p. 261). Campinha-Bacote (1999) refers to this stereotyping as a 'cultural blind spot' (p. 204). We, as nurses, could make the wrong assumption that there are no cultural differences or variations that could be barriers to care, and that everyone thinks, acts and feels the same way as we do. This would be a very ethnocentric view of the world, and would severely limit our ability to provide individualised care to patients and clients. Therefore, in Case study 5.4, Suri is no more a product merely of her ethnic group, in the same way as Paul and Rick are not merely stereotypes of a homosexual relationship. It can be difficult for a loving, long-standing homosexual partnership to be accepted by a society which has been acclimatised to believe that homosexual men are promiscuous and not committed to any one partner. This is clearly not the case with Paul and Rick.

The importance of a **cultural assessment** is crucial to Sue using her **cultural skills** and her **cultural sensitivity**. Sue is an active partner in the care that Paul needs and, as Papadopoulos and Lees (2002) say, this involves 'a process of facilitation, advocacy and negotiation that can only be achieved on a foundation of trust, respect and empathy' (p. 261). Paul and Rick trust Sue and feel respected by her and she, in turn, is empathetic towards them. This allows her to be in a position where she can be a negotiator and advocate on their behalf.

Sue used many **cultural skills** in her negotiations with Paul, Rick and their families. In some cases, cultural skills can include the problems of communicating when language barriers are present. Martinez (1994, cited in Kim-Godwin, Clarke and Barton 2001) gives a very emotive and distressing example of when communication was ineffective because of language difficulties. The example related the experience of a Mexican woman who went to the emergency room thinking she was still pregnant. She was worried about her unborn child's lack of obvious growth and she was speaking in Spanish. Two months earlier she had miscarried during a visit to another emergency room and she never understood that her baby had died and she was no longer pregnant, because nobody at that hospital had spoken her language. This clearly demonstrates the level of distressing miscommunication that can happen when language barriers exist. In these cases, nurses often use gestures or non-verbal communication, which can be limited in their effectiveness. In addition, they can use interpreters, which can also be inappropriate. The Royal College of Nursing (1994, cited in Holland and Hogg 2001) report on

the problems of using untrained interpreters as being:
- ➤ inaccurate translation;
- ➤ bias and distortion;
- ➤ lack of confidentiality;
- ➤ no understanding of the role;
- ➤ no explanation of cultural differences;
- ➤ personal unsuitability.

It is important for nurses to understand the potential problems that there can be in using interpreters. Confidential or personal information should not be shared with family members or friends, and this is particularly inappropriate where English speaking relatives of a different gender, or children, are used to explain about medical problems or ask about symptoms. Using someone who is not a family member can be a problem due to a potential lack of confidentiality, distortion or bias, and within any cultural group, others who speak the same language may be considered inappropriate due to their different backgrounds. Inaccurate translation and miscommunication should be avoided at all costs if effective communication is seen as 'getting the right message to the right people at the right time with the intended effect' (Ratzan 2001), or as 'clear, unambiguous two-way constructive exchanges, without distortion of the message between what is given and what is received' (Ewles and Simnett 2003).

It is also important for nurses to understand that there can be cultural differences in how patients express their symptoms, and this can make diagnosis difficult and symptoms can be misunderstood. For example, in mental health, terms such as the following can be used to describe feelings of depression (WONCA Special Interest Group 2004):
- ➤ feeling hot;
- ➤ sinking heart;
- ➤ gas;
- ➤ brain exploding;
- ➤ my head is empty;
- ➤ broken body;
- ➤ fatigued;
- ➤ heaviness in the head;
- ➤ biting sensation all over the body.

As WONCA (2004) say, 'A patient's cultural background will influence the metaphor they choose to describe psychological distress and their mood state. The side effects and dosage of antidepressant agents may also depend on ethnicity.'

It is important for nurses to try to understand a person's situation from that person's perspective. In an American study of African American older people, Shellman (2004) says that it is important to encourage the use of patient stories, narratives and reminiscences to try to find out about people's experiences. This is essential in carrying out culturally competent care. Patients often say that nobody has ever asked them a similar question before. There are stories of discrimination, and how people have coped with it, which can help to explain their fear or anticipation of discrimination and the ongoing hurt that this has caused. If nurses are not aware of this, they again can fail to care for people in a culturally competent manner. Crigger and Holcomb (2007) also stress the importance of providing culturally sensitive and ethnically responsive care and how this can influence ethical decision making and enhance multi-culturalism in developing nations. These same principles of nursing care, being ethically sound and culturally appropriate, should exist everywhere in the world.

A final point is that, within any particular culture, there can be senior members of the community who are influential and crucial to individual decision making. In an American study into the Hmong culture in the Central Valley of California, Mochel and Bauer (2005) say the Shamans are the key influential people in their communities and their perspective needs to be understood as they are the gateway to the rest of their community. In some families from the Indian subcontinent, the man's mother is a very influential person and a daughter-in-law will often defer decisions about her care, or that of her children, to her mother-in-law. If a nurse, midwife or health visitor is unaware of this, they can fail to understand how decisions about personal care are made within the family and all advice proves ineffectual.

The effectiveness of intercultural communication relies on a nurse's ability to be culturally knowledgeable, skilled and sensitive.

THOUGHTS FOR YOUR PRACTICE

- How do you ensure that your contacts with patients and clients enhance your ongoing cultural knowledge?
- Can you think of ways in which your assessment of patients could become more culturally focused?
- How could you share this developing knowledge with colleagues and students?

- Identify a situation where there was a language barrier with a patient or client. Could your communication have been enhanced in any way? If so what have you learnt for future practice?
- How can you increase the use of cultural skills within your practice?
- How can you become more culturally sensitive in your nursing care?
- In relation to your own personal norms and prejudices, are there any groups of people that you find it difficult to relate to? If so, who?
- Try to think of ways in which you can increase your cultural knowledge, understanding and acceptance of patients or clients whom you care for in your professional role.

SUMMARY – LINKS TO COMPASSION AND CARING

By focusing on diversity and cultural competence, this chapter has hopefully given you further insight into what it means to deliver compassionate care. Unfortunately, inequalities in health persist within and between countries, and some people do not have the same access to healthcare as others. Some individuals are more likely to be marginalised or socially excluded and this has the potential to negatively impact on their health. It is essential that nurses value difference and diversity, and that they see people who are different to them as an asset and not a problem. We need to understand who might be socially excluded and disadvantaged in order to practise in a socially inclusive way.

Once we have identified people who have different needs and different cultural norms and values to ourselves, we then need to strive to be as culturally competent as possible. This involves understanding different cultural identities, being culturally aware and culturally sensitive, and developing our cultural knowledge and skills. Codes of conduct for nursing should focus on equality and anti-discriminative practice. An example from the UK is from the Nursing and Midwifery Council's (NMC) code of conduct for nurses, which states that 'you must not discriminate in any way against those in your care and that you must demonstrate a personal and professional commitment to equality and diversity' (NMC 2008).

As Chen and Starosta (1997) say, cultural communication competence involves intercultural awareness, which is the 'ability to understand cultural similarities and differences and this is enhanced and buffered by cultural sensitivity' (p. 15), which is demonstrated by 'a positive attitude to cultural differences and a demonstration of flexibility in behaviour' (p. 15).

It is important for us to realise that we are all essentially ethnocentric. We adhere to our own set of cultural norms and values and that gives us our cultural identity. This cultural identity reflects who we are and what we believe is right or wrong. We are then ethnocentric in believing that everyone should think the way we do and make similar decisions about their lives and lifestyles. Unfortunately, this can lead us to believe that others' choices in life, or their lifestyles, are less valid than our own. Therefore, we start to stereotype and judge people based on our own assumptions and values. We are who we are, and in our personal lives we might struggle with accepting certain groups in society, yet as nurses we have to be able to provide professional and culturally competent care, which does not reflect our prejudices. If we do not, we cannot be compassionate and caring within our personal nursing practice.

REFERENCES

Alexis O, Chambers C. Exploring Alexis' model: valuing resources. Part 2. *Nursing Management*. 2003; **10**(5): 29–33.

Ali S, Atkin K. *Primary Healthcare and South Asian Populations: meeting the challenges*. Oxford: Radcliffe Medical Press; 2004.

Baxter C. *Managing Diversity and Inequality in Healthcare*. Edinburgh: Bailliere Tindall; 2001.

Black D. A doctor looks at health economics. In: Robinson J, Elkan R, editors. *Health Needs Assessment*. London: Churchill Livingstone; 1996.

Bradshaw J. The concept of social need. *New Society*. 1972; **30**(3): 640–3.

Campinha-Bacote J. A model and instrument for addressing cultural competence in healthcare. *J Nurs Educ*. 1999; **38**(5): 203–7.

Campinha-Bacote J. The process of cultural competence in the delivery of healthcare services: a model of care. *J Transcult Nurs*. 2002; **13**(3):181–4.

Chambers C, Alexis O. Creating an inclusive environment for Black and ethnic nurses. *BJN*. 2004; **13**(22): 1355–8.

Chen G, Starosta W. A review of the concept of intercultural sensitivity. *Human Communication*. 1997; 1(1): 1–16.

Chen G, Starosta W. The development and validation of the intercultural communication sensitivity scale. *Human Communication*. 2000; **3**: 1–35.

Cortis J. Culture, values and racism: application to nursing. *Int Nurs Rev*. 2003; **50**(1): 55–64.

Crigger N, Holcomb L. Practical strategies for providing culturally sensitive, ethical care in developing nations. *J Transcult Nurs*. 2007; **18**(1): 70–6.

Department of Health. *Saving Lives: our healthier nation*. Cm 4386. London: Department of Health; 1999.

Department of Health. *National Service Framework for Coronary Heart Disease*. London: Department of Health; 2000.

Department of Health. *National Service Framework for Older People*. London: Department of Health; 2001.

Department of Health. *Women's Mental Health in the Mainstream*. London: Department of Health; 2002.

Department of Health. *The National Service Framework for Long-Term Conditions*. London: Department of Health; 2005.

Ewles L, Simnett I. *Promoting Health: a practical guide*. 5th ed. London: Balliere Tindall; 2003.

Galdas P, Cheater F, Marshall P. Men and health-seeking behaviour: literature review. *J Adv Nurs*. 2005; **49**(6): 616–23.

Gerrish K, Papadopoulos I. Transcultural competence: the challenge for nurse education. *BJN*. 1999; **8**(21): 1453–7.

Hilgenberg E, Schlickau J. Building transcultural knowledge through intercollegiate collaboration. *J Transcult Nurs*. 2002; **13**(3): 241–7.

Holland K, Hogg C. *Cultural Awareness in Nursing and Health Care*. London: Arnold Publishers; 2001.

Home Office. *The UK Human Rights Act*. London: Home Office; 1998.

Husain F. *Cultural Competence in Family Support*. London: National Family and Parenting Institute; 2005.

Jandt F. *Intercultural Communication: an introduction*. 3rd ed. London: Sage Publications; 2001.

Kim-Godwin Y, Clarke P, Barton L. A model for the delivery of cultural competent community care. *J Adv Nurs*. 2001: **35**(6): 918–25.

Mochel M, Bauer R. Chronic illness and Hmong Shamans. *J Transcult Nurs*. 2005; **16**(2): 150–4.

Nursing and Midwifery Council. *The Code: standards of conduct, performance and ethics for nurses and midwives*. London: Nursing and Midwifery Council; 2008.

Papadopoulos I, Lees S. Developing culturally competent researchers. *J Adv Nurs*. 2002; **37**(3): 258–64.

Papadopoulos I, Tilki M, Taylor G. *Transcultural Care: a guide for healthcare professionals*. Trowbridge: Mark Allen Publishers; 1998.

Ratzan S. Health literacy: communication for the public good. *Health Promot Int*. 2001; **16**(2): 207–14.

Robotham A, Sheldrake D. *Health Visiting: specialist and higher level practice*. London: Churchill Livingstone; 2000.

Shaw M, Davey Smith G, Dorling D. Health inequalities and New Labour: how the promises compare with real progress. *BMJ*. 2005; **330**(7498): 1016–21.

Shellman J. 'Nobody ever asked me before': understanding life experiences of African American elders. *J Transcult Nurs*. 2004; **15**(4): 308–16.

Silver H. Social exclusion: comparative analysis of Europe and Middle East youth. *Middle East Youth Initiative Working Paper*; 2007.

The Salvation Army. *The Seeds of Exclusion*. London: The Salvation Army; 2008.

Thompson N. *Anti-discriminatory Practice*. 3rd ed. Basingstoke: Palgrave; 2001.

Thompson N. *Promoting Equality: challenging discrimination and oppression*. 2nd ed. Basingstoke: Palgrave MacMillan; 2003.

WONCA Special Interest Group in Psychiatry and Neurology. *Culturally Sensitive Depression Guideline*. London: WONCA; 2004.

World Health Organization. *Closing the Gap in a Generation: health equity through action on the social determinants of health*. Geneva: World Health Organization; 2008.

CHAPTER 6

Choice and priorities

Overview of the chapter

Key theme one – choice
- Case study
- Discussion
- Do we genuinely understand the meaning of working in partnership with our patients and clients?
- Case study
- Discussion
- Thoughts for your practice
- How can we increase patient participation in making choices about their care?
- Case study
- Discussion
- Thoughts for your practice

Key theme two – priorities
- Case study
- Discussion
- Do we know what the priorities of our patients and clients are?
- Case study
- Discussion
- Thoughts for your practice
- Do we genuinely base our practice around patient and client priorities?
- Case study
- Discussion
- Thoughts for your practice
- Summary – links to compassion and caring
- References

OVERVIEW OF THE CHAPTER

A recurrent theme that has emerged throughout our consideration of each aspect of compassionate care, so far, is the importance of meeting patient or client needs by adopting a person-centred approach. If we are serious in wanting to meet these needs, this will involve working in partnership with those for whom we care. As nurses we need to support people to actively participate in trying to make choices about their care a reality. We need to ensure that we prioritise what they would prioritise in relation to their care, wherever possible. This process may well pose dilemmas for nurses as prioritising patient needs could conflict with resources available and practitioner priorities. Therefore, this chapter will look at these issues in more depth in order to ensure that there is a humane and caring approach to practice.

KEY THEME ONE – CHOICE

CASE STUDY 6.1

Sally had been visiting Bob and Betty at home for some time in her role as nurse coordinator of Bob's care. She felt that she knew them quite well and she knew when something was worrying them. Bob was very close to death from lung cancer. He had never smoked, but had worked for many years in an environment that would have been considered unsafe nowadays because of the high levels of asbestos. Neither of them dwelt on the unfairness of his disease. He was only 70 and should have had many more years to live. As a couple they were exceptionally close and Sally felt very sad for them, especially when she saw how strong Betty was trying to be for Bob.

When she went in today she could see that something was on their minds. Bob was looking frailer every day, but as usual they both greeted her with a smile. Their home was full of Christmas cards; they had a large loving family and a lot of friends and were very much loved and appreciated by a lot of people. Sally admired the cards and asked how things were today. Bob was struggling to breathe and looking very cyanosed, and he looked to Betty to say what he obviously wanted to say.

Betty started very tentatively by saying how much they appreciated the care that had been available to them at home. They felt very much cared for and appreciated everything that Sally and the team were doing to help ease Bob's final days. However, they knew how little time he had left; this would be his last Christmas and they wanted it to be as special as possible. Their family would be popping in throughout the Christmas period, but Bob was easily tired and needed to have time to rest between visits from them. They wanted to spend as much of the precious time they had together just on their own and being with each other. Their families understood this and a plan had been worked out for who would visit when, and for how long. This left the majority of the time free for Bob and Betty to just be together.

Sally could see that there was something more they wanted to say and asked how they wanted the nursing side of Bob's care to fit in with their plans over the holidays, because there were plans for various people to visit over that time. Betty said that they really did not want any visits over the next few days. They felt that they understood enough about Bob's analgesia to keep his pain under control. His oxygen supplies were already there and they felt that his other care needs could be managed by them or left for a while.

Sally's immediate feelings were of concern for Bob's welfare. He was a seriously ill man whose needs could become very acute and distressing very fast and she did not want either of them to suffer any more than they already were. However, she could see how important their last days together were to them both. It must be very intrusive and disruptive to have visits from care agencies all the time. Sally smiled reassuringly, made these points and said that as long as they were happy with the situation at any given point then nobody would visit. However, if that changed, and they were worried, then she would be available on her mobile and would make sure that problems were solved or alleviated as they arose. She also asked if she could phone a couple of times a day, and they arranged mutually convenient times for the calls. She could see their anxiety starting to ease when they realised that she was not offended and, indeed, understood their point of view, while still feeling that the care that might be needed could still be available.

Discussion

This situation created a dilemma for Sally. She was trying to balance the nursing needs that she knew Bob had with trying to honour their personal choice about what they felt they wanted at this time. She was concerned that his care might be compromised and wanted to reach some negotiated agreement about how contact could be maintained from both sides. It is always difficult to ensure that patients and clients actually make an **informed decision** based on real knowledge about the problems they might face. Bob and Betty just wanted to have time on their own, but they might have failed to appreciate emergencies that can develop when someone is as ill as Bob. This would have needed a full and frank discussion, which is not fully represented in the case study discussion. Sally was using all her interpersonal skills and clinical decision making, including:

➤ assessment skills;
➤ tact and diplomacy;
➤ advanced decision making;
➤ advanced problem solving;
➤ empathy and understanding of their needs and priorities;
➤ working in partnership;
➤ verbal and non-verbal skills about what was said and not said;
➤ negotiation and real-choice options;
➤ anticipation of needs based on real knowledge of their situation;
➤ use of her therapeutic long-standing relationship;
➤ coordination skills with other agencies.

In their Norwegian based study, Hauge and Heggen (2008) make the point that by moving into a care environment, choices can be more limited and many compromises have to be made. They say that relationships can be enforced and privacy and control can be lost. This could have been the case with Bob and Betty, who were still in their own home. Choices could have been limited by Bob's health needs and the services that were available. It is important that nurses work within the boundaries of what is reasonable and realistic in a resource constrained health service and patient choices cannot always be honoured. However, it would also be easy for Sally to have made decisions purely from her own professional perspective, without trying to make compromises, based on Bob and Betty's choices. Their privacy and sense of control could have been severely compromised by Sally providing the service that she normally would have given, rather than providing a service that met their individual needs. It is important for nurses to realise that people who have been in long-term partnerships probably have an intimate relationship that could be compromised if only one partner needs care. At this point, partners can be separated as their care needs become too difficult to manage within one environment, be it at home or in more formal care settings. This can be an impossible problem to solve. However, if nurses have used all their problem-solving skills to try not to separate partners, and if they are aware and sensitive about how this separation might be affecting both parties, they can be sure that they are providing care that is as good as possible within the services constraints that inevitably exist.

Nurses need to ensure that patients, carers and clients feel that they can take an active part in making choices about their care. Some people do not have the confidence or the communication strategies to express their wishes. Some have been brought up not to question professional decision making and they feel that they have to accept what is offered. As the choices and expectations of different generations change, we as nurses need to be able to adapt to these changes.

A UK Department of Health report says that:

> Choice gives patients the power they need . . . Where patients find it difficult to express preferences it is the role of staff to take steps to ensure that patients can benefit from greater choice. Choice in public services is sometimes presented as the preoccupation of the wealthy and the educated, yet the evidence shows that it is the poorest and least educated who most desire greater choice. (DOH 2008, p. 38)

It is the nurse's role to try to encourage patient participation and work in partnership with those in their care, to encourage communication about their choices and to ensure that choices are real and not merely rhetoric.

Do we genuinely understand the meaning of working in partnership with our patients and clients?

CASE STUDY 6.2

Amanda really enjoyed working with people with learning disabilities and had chosen this option right from the start of her nursing career. She knew that many people shied away from people who were 'different' and also that communicating with her clients was often difficult for those with no experience of talking to people who expressed themselves in different ways. She found this to be a particularly interesting part of her role and finding alternative ways to bond with her clients was an ongoing and stimulating part of communicating with them.

Today was busy as usual and she knew that Pat wanted to buy a present for her friend Jane. Amanda often went out for a walk with Pat, but it would take longer if it involved buying a present too. She knew that this would be a time-consuming activity, and one that she could much more easily accomplish by buying something herself for Pat to give to Jane. However, it was important for Pat to interact with as wide a range of people as possible. She had very few friends, so choosing a present herself was very important to her.

Having found out that Pat thought Jane would really like some new earrings, Amanda took Pat to a shop that sold inexpensive earrings and had a wide variety of choice. Pat was overwhelmed by all the pretty, sparkly earrings on display. She thought that they were beautiful. Amanda asked Pat what colour earrings she thought that Jane might like, whether she wanted long or short ones and how much she wanted to spend. Having decided that long sparkly blue ones were in keeping with Jane's way of dressing, they set about trying to find ones that Pat thought Jane would like best. After a great deal of deliberation Pat chose a pair that were not very expensive and there was a matching pendant that Pat could buy too, within her budget, and Amanda drew her attention to this. Pat was really pleased with this choice. Amanda could see that Pat's attention was drawn to some other purple glass earrings and she knew that Pat loved purple. Amanda looked at the price and saw that they were on discount and could actually be bought, still within Pat's budget. Amanda picked up the purple earrings and held them against Pat's ears and moved a mirror so Pat could see how they would look on her. Her face lit up and she said 'beautiful'. Amanda said to Pat that she did indeed look beautiful and said that she had enough money to buy these too. Pat was so excited that she started to jump up and down. People in the shop started to look alarmed and move away, but Pat was so excited that she did not notice. Just then a little girl, about five years of age, pulled on Pat's sleeve and said, 'I think those look lovely on you'. Her mother came from behind the counter and agreed, then smiled at Pat and asked if she would like them to be put in a pretty box. Pat nodded and gave her the blue pendant and earrings and it was clear she wanted to wear the purple ones.

Despite the developing queue to pay, the owner of the shop patiently explained how much money she needed from the large number of coins that Pat had. Amanda wished everyone was so understanding and accepting of those who had learning disabilities. She felt renewed by her faith in people and was really glad that she had spent the extra time in the shop that Pat had needed to make the decision about the present for her friend.

Discussion

Amanda is clearly working in partnership with Pat. She understands what is important to Pat, how some people with whom she comes into contact might judge her, and, even more essentially, what is important to her. Amanda is a busy practitioner who knows that she could sort out the present buying much faster if she took more control of the situation. However, it is important that it is Pat's choice and she makes the decision; Amanda is there really just to facilitate this. This case study clearly demonstrates a high level of sensitive partnership working.

Papadopoulos and Lees (2002) say that 'partnership demands that power relationships are challenged and that real choices are offered' (p. 261). Amanda was very clearly passing over power and the decision making to Pat in order that Pat could make the decisions herself.

Amanda is not expecting Pat to comply with decisions that have already been made; the partnership she is demonstrating indicates that their relationship is based firmly on concordance. Concordance involves a negotiation between equals based on a therapeutic relationship, which will be discussed in more detail in Chapter 7. Cuff (in Burley, *et al.* 1997) says that a therapeutic relationship involves the sharing in partnership of:

➤ information
➤ planning and decision making
➤ responsibility
➤ control and power.

Wallis (2007) writes about a young man living with a life-limiting and debilitating disease, who wanted to experience sexual activity before he died. The hospice facilitated this in his own home despite the fact that they were aware that he really wanted an emotionally fulfilling relationship and he could be disappointed with just sexual activity. The fact that he wanted to make his own choice was seen as paramount. A senior member of church felt that the decision to allow this to take place demonstrated true humanity and compassion. His disability prevented him from independently making his own choice and the hospice respected his autonomy and his right to make his own decision. This young man felt empowered by his part in the decision-making process and said, 'My experience taught me a lot and gave me a sense of normality – to a degree. It also helped me to realise that I could make things happen if I really wanted them enough' (Wallis 2007, p. 4). Although the experience lacked the emotional element that he wanted so much and he did not necessarily want to repeat the experience, it was of paramount importance to him to feel in control of his own destiny and life experiences. Therefore, the therapeutic relationships that facilitated this did involve partnership in relation to information, planning, decision making, responsibility, control and power.

Both Case study 6.2 and the experience that Wallis writes about demonstrate concordance, which is evidenced by respect for the patient's perspective, promotion of patient autonomy and self-determination. Therefore, the patient or client is actively engaged in the decision making. Problem solving, negotiation and partnership are key elements of working in partnership. Hornby and Atkins (2000) say that certain attitudes are essential for working in partnership; for example, reciprocity, flexibility and professional integrity. Again, both in the case study and in Wallis' article, power and control were devolved in a reciprocal manner, there was flexibility and the professionals involved demonstrated professional integrity.

Working in partnership is not always easy and relies heavily on the nature and strength of the relationship between nurse and patient or client.

> For older people who are not yet self-agents in their care, providing the clinical and social environments for them to grow and learn is essential. The way to do this is not to assume we know what they want to learn, but rather to offer a participative partnership that facilitates their control of 'what' and how it is offered. (Koch, Jenkin and Kralik 2004, p. 490)

It is not just older people who have difficulty working in partnership in making decisions about their care. It is important to realise that there is a clear power imbalance when a person is receiving care from others, and possibly has less knowledge about their health condition and what services are available. People need to feel empowered in order to make choices. Wilkinson (2007) says that people should have access to knowledge of care choices and the treatment success from different people's personal experiences, as well as their rights of complaint and how they can take part in satisfaction surveys. There are new options that are becoming more accepted by patients and healthcare professionals, such as some complementary therapies and exercise programmes rather than medication, but patients might be less aware of these options.

Having discussed the importance of working in partnership with patients and clients and what it actually means, it is now important to discuss ways in which we can increase patient participation in the choices about their care.

THOUGHTS FOR YOUR PRACTICE

- Can you think of a time when a patient's choices were compromised?
- On reflection, do you think that more choices were available?
- If so, how could you have encouraged those choices to have been more real?
- Have there been times when you have not been able to meet someone's choices, when you would have liked to facilitate this?
- If so, how did you explain this to the person involved?
- How could you further enhance your ability to encourage patients to express their choices?
- How could you encourage others to challenge their own practice in this way?
- Do you feel that there are ways in which you could further decrease the power imbalance between you and your patients?
- How could you share your thoughts with others?
- Think of an example when your relationship with a patient has been truly concordant and one where it has not. What made the difference between the two situations?
- What have you learnt from this for future practice, and how can you share this with others?
- Can you think of ways in which you can develop your skills further in relation to working in partnership with patients and clients?
- Is there anything about partnership working that you have learnt that could be adopted by your practice team?

How can we increase patient participation in choices about their care?

CASE STUDY 6.3

Zack was restless and angry. He never knew where this anger came from and was aware that the reason he was in the forensic mental health unit was because anger took him over, unexpectedly, at times. He never knew how he might react when these intense feelings hit him. He had harmed someone in the past during one of his bouts of anger. His sentence was to be carried out here in the forensic unit, rather than in prison, because it was felt that his problems were due to mental illness.

Zack did not want to hurt anyone ever again, and it was obviously safer for other people for him to be here. Although he felt that he was in a therapeutic environment and not just a custodial one, this sometimes made his lack of freedom more pronounced. He did not have choices about how he spent his time and the system determined what time he got up, when and what he ate, when he was allowed to have exercise and when he went to bed. He felt like a caged animal with no rights, no choices and no ability to make decisions for himself.

Discussion

Zack was clearly in a situation where he had to be contained to protect the safety of others. Therefore, he had to comply with what the system dictated and could take no part in decisions that involved him in most areas of his life. Other people might feel the same way despite the fact that they are not legally required to be somewhere. For example, there are many people who are not able to care for themselves at home and, therefore, are cared for in a more formal setting. They might also lack many of the choices that Zack is lacking.

Older people with mental health problems might be in residential care, but their privacy should be respected as should their priorities at all times. Knocking on the door to someone's private room should not just be a formality where the nurse knocks and walks straight in. The individual concerned should have the opportunity to answer and invite the nurse to enter, or ask them to wait a moment, in the same way as we do in our own homes. A nurse should always respect what someone wants to be called rather than make assumptions. They might not want to be called by their first name, or they might want their occupation in life to be recognised by the terms Father, Reverend, Major or Doctor, and this again should be respected. Other people might want a choice about whether they have a bath or a shower, how often this is, and when it takes place. As long as there is a bath or shower available, staffing levels allow and hygiene is being maintained, then these choices should be available. However, too often decisions are made about what is easier for the service, despite the fact that choice is possible and would not be disruptive within the environment in which the person is being cared for. Mealtimes can be another time when no choice is available. Some people might choose to miss breakfast and have a lie in, and this would not be detrimental to their health. Others might not feel well enough to eat a meal, but might be able to tolerate a milkshake or a smoothie, and this could be possible within the resources available. In order for any of these things to take place, people have to be given options and genuinely asked what they would prefer in order to make informed choice a reality.

As nurses, it is essential to realise how important choice is in relation to quality of life and what it means to individuals. Bowling and Gabriel (2007), in their study of older people in the UK, highlight 'health' as a key aspect of what quality of life means to individual older people. They found that people valued choices in life and saw these as 'empowerment, freedom, social participation and doing what they wanted to do' (p. 844). In a Taiwanese study, Yu-Ching, Ruey-Hsia and Shu-Hui (2006) supported this and found that older people in nursing homes said that empowering care was the most important predictor of quality of life. Choice is central to empowered care and this will be discussed further in Chapter 7.

As nurses, we face many dilemmas in nursing care, some of which surround the emotive areas of end-of-life and resuscitation choices. Dying with dignity is something we would all aspire to, and it is likely that we would see having choices about decisions in our final days as central to a 'good death'. We cannot predict how or when we will die in most cases – all we know is that our lives are finite. The point at which death becomes inevitable might not be immediate and might come at a point where we are unable to make choices for ourselves. Therefore, we would hope that nurses who are involved in our care would be sensitive, empathetic and respectful of us, and would be actively trying to protect our dignity. Someone who is in a permanent vegetative state, and has been for 10 years, might never have wanted their lives prolonged. However, it is impossible for someone who is unable to respond to make a choice about ending their life, or what measures should be taken if their condition worsens. This could involve not actively treating infections or increasing medical interventions, or not resuscitating someone. There have been key cases, widely reported by the media, around not prolonging life, which have involved withholding food or fluids. Some nurses and healthcare professionals have questioned the humanity of this; there is a narrow line between not prolonging life and actively helping someone to die. The British Medical Association (BMA 2002) has produced guidelines in relation to decision making for resuscitation and this emphasises the importance of a partnership approach involving the patient, their close friends and relatives and the multi-professional team caring for the person.

> You and your doctor will decide whether CPR should be attempted if you have a cardiopulmonary arrest. The healthcare team looking after you will look at all the medical issues, including whether CPR is likely to be able to restart your heart and breathing if they stop, and for how long. It is beneficial to

attempt resuscitation if it might prolong your life in a way that you can enjoy. Sometimes, however, restarting people's heart and breathing leaves them with a severe disability or only prolongs their suffering. Prolonging life in these circumstances is not always beneficial. Your wishes are very important in deciding whether resuscitation can benefit you, and the healthcare team will want to know what you think. If you want, your close friends and family can be involved in discussions. In most cases, doctors and their patients agree about treatment where there has been good communication. (BMA 2002, p. 5)

We cannot always assume that all relatives or next of kin are striving for what the patient would have wanted, although this is often the case.

In order for compassionate and caring decisions to be made in relation to end-of-life issues, it is important for nurses to make sure that decisions are not based on their own beliefs and principles, but on an ethical basis that is as objective as possible. Nurses should aim to maximise and honour a person's choices and bear in mind that patients should, whenever possible, be treated as partners in any decisions concerning their needs and priorities.

THOUGHTS FOR YOUR PRACTICE

- How do you involve patients and clients in decisions about their care?
- How do you ensure that you offer as great a range of choices as possible?
- Do you feel that there are times when you put service needs before the choices of patients or clients?
- How do you work in partnership with people to find out what quality of life means to them?
- Do you ever feel that your own personal beliefs influence the way you present choices to patients or clients?
- How can you try to identify when this happens and how can you refocus possible choices around the patient's agenda?

KEY THEME TWO – PRIORITIES

CASE STUDY 6.4

Katy had spent the whole morning rushing around. She really enjoyed the diversity of her school nursing role, but there was a lot to fit into the relatively short day, when children and young people were more available because they were in school. She had been supervising an immunisation session that morning. She was trying to ease anxiety levels among the young people, who were likely to try to do the opposite, as well as ensuring the session was as efficient as possible. This was always a challenge.

She had then driven the short distance to another school to see Adam, who had been diagnosed with diabetes a few months beforehand. Adam was eight years old and he was already able to use the blood glucose monitoring machine and understand the readings to a level that he could work out the insulin dose he needed. She thought that he had done very well in the circumstances. He was able to give his own injections, but he had not got enough confidence yet to give the injections on his own and nobody at the school felt able to take on this role. Katy was genuinely impressed with how much Adam had achieved as he also had to cope with accepting the fact that he had a health condition that would be with him for life. However, she felt that she was there more as a reassurance than as a nurse. She knew that soon Adam would have enough confidence to do this on his own, but, although she saw this as a priority, at the moment the daily visits to the school were putting quite a pressure on the school nursing service. She was also aware that there were increasing pressures on the service including more children developing long-term conditions, more mental health issues among young people and younger children, a rising teenage pregnancy rate, increased incidence of sexually transmitted infections in the school-age population and more children with special needs. The service was under immense pressure, and priorities would have to be made from the service point of view, which would not necessarily be based on the needs of the children and young people in schools she covered.

Discussion

This case study highlights the dilemma that a nursing service has in trying to meet an increasingly wide diversity of needs within a financially constrained healthcare environment. Adam has done very well to progress to the point where he was able to work out his own insulin dose, draw it up into a syringe and inject it himself. Understandably, he is still lacking confidence, and Katy might have been visiting to carry out more of the care herself if he had not become independent so fast. The fact that he is largely self-caring means that her skills are not needed to such a great extent. However, this means that it is less easy to justify her nursing time in Adam's situation. Her experience enabled her to realise that his developing confidence might be easily damaged and that spending time at this point was not only a priority for him, but for the school nursing service, because he would become totally independent much more quickly.

In the previous section, we discussed the importance of offering choice to patients and clients. However, the reality of healthcare provision is that choices need to be balanced with service resources, targets and priorities. Therefore, in the following section, we will be discussing whether we know what our patients' and clients' priorities are and whether we actually base our practice around these.

Do we know what the priorities of our patients and clients are?

CASE STUDY 6.5

Brian had known for some time that his drinking was out of control. He was aware of what an important part alcohol was playing in his life. If he was not actually drinking, he was either recovering from the effect of his last drink or thinking about when his next drink would be, sometimes both at the same time. This was not going to be a long-term solution to his loneliness and distress following the death of his beloved wife Val. They had always been so close and had done everything together, and her illness had been so sudden and so short that he had found himself on his own before he had really known what was happening. He knew that Val would be very sad if she could see how his life was at the moment, and he knew that he owed it to her, as well as himself, to stop drinking before he lost his job and probably his home.

He had made an appointment to see Hamed, the Occupational Health Nurse, with some trepidation. After all, Hamed was employed by the company too, and he really was not sure about whether this could be a confidential discussion or not. Brian knew that he was not putting anybody else at risk within his workplace by his drinking, but he was damaging his own health.

Hamed greeted Brian in an informal manner and immediately explained that any conversation between them would be confidential, unless there were any safety issues involved, in which case they would discuss a way forward that would hopefully solve the immediate situation. Only in extreme circumstances would Hamed have to report a situation to someone within the company.

Brian immediately felt more relaxed. He had met Hamed only on the odd occasion before, but had never talked to him on a one-to-one basis. He knew that Hamed was Muslim and, therefore, was unlikely to drink at all, but he felt that Hamed was someone who was unlikely to judge him for the fact that he was drinking.

Hamed said that he could see that Brian was unhappy and Brian told him about how much he missed Val. To his embarrassment he started to cry, but Hamed carried on talking gently to him about the person Val had been, what their relationship had been like and how he was coping with his immense loss. Brian knew then that Hamed would understand and told him how worried he was by his drinking. Hamed asked how much he was drinking and did not seem shocked by the reply. Brian told him how much he wanted to stop drinking, but that he needed help. Hamed was reassuring and said that it was not uncommon for people to develop negative coping strategies at times of stress or bereavement. He gave him some numbers to ring for an alcohol service and for counselling and then said that he would like to keep in contact too, so that he has someone to support him in the work environment. Brian felt so relieved, not only because help and support were available and he thought the counselling was a good idea, but also because Hamed was prepared to support him while he was at work. He felt that he really would be able to fight his need for drink with appropriate support.

Discussion

When he went to see Hamed, Brian's priorities were about being able to trust him. He needed him to be non-judgemental, sensitive and supportive, but he also needed the conversation to be confidential. Hamed was aware of this and he started off by discussing where confidentiality started and ended. Nurses need to be aware of the importance of having this conversation at the start of their relationship with someone, because wrong assumptions can be made. A patient can assume that everything will remain confidential, despite the fact that they have raised issues that put others at risk. If a nurse, midwife or health visitor discusses how they have to protect the safety of vulnerable people and children and therefore confidentiality cannot be protected in situations where there is obvious risk, then everyone is clear from the start. In occupational health settings, a nurse has to be able to make difficult decisions about the safety of others. If Brian's drinking was putting others at risk, because he was driving or operating machinery, Hamed would have needed to take this into account in relation to the confidentiality of their discussions. Therefore, the fact that Hamed raised this at the start of the conversation had the effect of reassuring Brian and made it possible for their future conversations to be based on an informed understanding.

Hamed then started to develop a trusting and supportive relationship with Brian. His non-judgemental and supportive approach was key to Brian feeling that he could discuss his problems openly, including his use of alcohol as a negative coping strategy. Therefore, Brian could start to trust Hamed. This trustworthiness also involved Brian knowing that Hamed was operating in an evidence-based way, and was knowledgeable about up-to-date services, treatments and options. A trusting professional relationship is also based on a nurse being professional in appearance and attitude, which is important for patient confidence and helps to reduce worry and concern. This was clearly evident in the developing relationship between Brian and Hamed.

Hamed's relationship with Brian was based strongly on psychological support, good communication, empathy, sensitivity and kindness. He was aware of available resources and could coordinate these in a way that was meaningful for Brian's situation. Hamed also stressed his accessibility and availability, and he offered ongoing support, which allowed Brian to feel that there would be continuity of care. He was clearly there to help Brian to achieve his goal in relation to coping with his use of alcohol. During their consultation, all of these components of care were based clearly on Brian's needs and priorities, without compromising Hamed's professional nursing practice.

This focus on patient, carer and client priorities was clearly identified in an Australian study by Gullick and Shimadry (2008), who asked for patient and client views on their experiences to improve quality of care. They used the Picker criteria of the nine valued domains of healthcare (Coulter 2006), which are:

➤ fast access to reliable healthcare;

➤ effective treatment delivered by trustworthy staff;
➤ involvement in decisions, and respect for preferences;
➤ clear, comprehensible information throughout the journey;
➤ attention to physical and environmental needs;
➤ emotional support, empathy and respect;
➤ involvement of, and support for, family and carers;
➤ smooth transition to, and support for, self-care;
➤ continuity and coordination of care.

In their study, Gullick and Shimadry (2008) found that the three most positive dimensions, according to the patients and carers, had been fast access to reliable healthcare, effective treatment delivered by trustworthy staff and the involvement of, and support for, family and carers.

The most negative experiences had been in relation to lack of clear, comprehensible information, lack of coordination and continuity of care and lack of attention to physical and environmental needs. Exclusion from care planning, lack of partnership, lack of communication and consultation were particularly highlighted.

In Brian's situation, he was respected and involved in decisions about his care within a trusting and therapeutic relationship. Hamed communicated his understanding of how the loss of his wife had devastated Brian and had a negative impact on his health and lifestyle choices. Hamed had been accessible to Brian at a time when Brian felt able to discuss his situation, and had been emotionally supportive to him. Furthermore, Hamed offered him continuity of care via his ongoing relationship with Brian.

The importance of continuity of care is highlighted in a Canadian study by Haggerty, *et al.* (2003). Continuity is mainly viewed as the relationship between a single practitioner and a patient that extends beyond specific episodes of illness or disease. Continuity implies a sense of affiliation between patients and their practitioners, often expressed in terms of an implicit contract of loyalty by the patient and clinical responsibility by the provider. Two core elements are:
➤ care of an individual in how individual patients experience integration of services and coordination;
➤ care delivered over time, which can be variable.

Haggerty, *et al.* (2003) say that for continuity to exist both elements must be present, and care must be experienced as connected and coherent. This was clearly the case in Brian's situation and his priorities had been recognised and met by Hamed, who had been able to identify Brian's priorities since the beginning of their conversation.

THOUGHTS FOR YOUR PRACTICE

- How do you know what your patient's priorities are?
- How do you ensure that you focus on these throughout your conversations with patients and clients?
- Do you sometimes feel that time constraints and your clinical priorities take precedence over your patients' priorities?
- How can you ensure that your patients' priorities remain paramount within the care they receive?
- Do you have explicit discussions about the nature of confidentiality within conversations with patients and clients?
- Do you have these discussions early enough in your professional relationships with people to ensure that there is clarity for all concerned?
- If not, how do you need to build this into your practice in a different way?

Do we genuinely base our practice around patient and client priorities?

CASE STUDY 6.6

Jenny was lying in bed behind the screens feeling terrified. She had never had an operation before and she was on her own and was feeling more like a child than the 16-year-old that she actually was. She was on her own and just wanted her mum, but of course that was not possible because of the reason she was here. She had felt that a termination of her pregnancy was the only way out of her desperate situation, but now she was not so sure.

She had not told her parents about that terrible night and she had been in denial for some weeks once she had finally known that she was pregnant, so this was probably the last opportunity for her to have a termination. She had ultimately plucked up the courage to tell her doctor, who had made an urgent referral to the hospital. Everything had gone very quickly from there, and now here she was waiting for the operation to take place.

They had asked her if she was sure that this was the decision she wanted to make and she had been absolutely sure. After all, how could you keep a baby who was not born out of love or even passion, but from power and violence? She felt that it must have been in some way her fault, that she had been giving out the wrong signals and that, therefore, she alone should suffer the consequences. She had been drinking that evening, but not enough to dull her senses or her decision making. She had gone to the toilet and, on the way out of the bathroom, her way downstairs had been blocked by a group of boys who she knew from school. They were in the year above and she had always secretly fancied Rob, so it must have been her fault what had happened then. They were all laughing and joking as they pushed her and Rob into an empty bedroom. Rob looked at her and she knew that he had taken something more than alcohol, although he had been drinking quite a bit too. His eyes were vacant as he pushed her down on the bed and he just ignored her efforts to get off the bed or her attempts to make him stop. She tried being angry, pleading with him, hitting him and then just cried as she accepted the inevitable. He just walked out of the room afterwards and she heard the group laughing as they went down the stairs.

She had lain there, crying, for some time and then ran down the stairs, ignoring her friends who were asking if she was alright. She did not know how she had got home, but she did, and she ran straight up the stairs and had a shower, then a bath, then another shower, but nothing made her feel clean. In the days afterwards, she had become withdrawn from her friends, brushed off her parents' concerned questions and hoped that she would not get pregnant or start getting symptoms of a sexually transmitted infection. She knew that her parents would have wanted her to go to the police and she could not bear that – all the questions and humiliation and perhaps silent blame.

So here she was, alone and crying, when Fiona, the nurse who had admitted her that morning, came to say that it would not be long until she went up to theatre.

Fiona knew as soon as she saw Jenny that something was very wrong. It was a busy list and her priority was on ensuring that everyone was prepared and ready to go up to theatre at the allotted time. However, she could not ignore Jenny's distress and had felt from the time she had met her that something was wrong. Telling Jenny she would be back in a minute she went to speak to a colleague and then back to talk to Jenny.

When Fiona went home that night she could not stop thinking about her day and about Jenny. Having said to her colleague that she needed to spend some time with Jenny because she felt that she could be in the process of making the wrong decision by having a termination, she then spent a long time talking to Jenny. She postponed the operation for the day and then after hearing of her horrendous experience, she persuaded Jenny to try to tell her mother. Jenny's mother arrived very distressed at the fact that Jenny was in hospital at all, and she became more distressed when she heard what had happened to her. Although she was strong for Jenny at the time, she and her husband had needed support later in the day. Fiona had coordinated discussions with her doctor, who had come down at the end of the theatre list, and had been very supportive and sympathetic. With Jenny's consent, she had also phoned the police who had arrived in the form of a sensitive officer who specialised in domestic abuse and crimes of a sexual nature. By the end of the day, Jenny was managing a brief smile and actually gave Fiona a quick hug to thank her. She went home with her parents and Fiona carried on with all the usual ward demands of pre- and post-operative care. She knew that her colleagues had had to cope with all these demands with one less team member, which had put them under immense pressure, but as a team they felt that they had made the right decisions and focused on the right priorities during a day that had brought increased and unexpected challenges.

Discussion

Jenny's situation is very distressing, and the fact that she is just about to go to theatre for her termination when this case study takes place puts additional pressure on the situation as there are clear time constraints. Fiona needs to act immediately if she to prevent a termination talking place that might not be the decision that Jenny actually wants. This involves sensitive and dynamic decision making, problem solving and prioritisation. It would be very easy for Fiona to perceive Jenny's distress as pre-theatre stress and carry on prioritising the day's work, ensuring that everybody is prepared adequately for their operation on time. However, being a nurse involves being dynamic in changing situations and this means reprioritising as necessary. These decisions need to be made based on conflicting professional demands, and this should include balancing the priorities of different patients and clients.

Fiona needs to ensure that the ward priorities are met and this involves discussion with other team members. This allows her to find time in a busy ward situation to prioritise Jenny's needs. The team supports Fiona in redefining her priorities, but even in relation to Jenny herself there are conflicting priorities. Fiona needs to postpone Jenny's operation (ensuring that this is also what Jenny wants) and contact relevant personnel. She also needs to seek Jenny's consent to arrange additional support for her – primarily her mother in this case. If this was inappropriate then other members of the multi-professional team, such as a social worker or a member of the clergy, might be acceptable to her. Social and medical needs all have to be balanced alongside organisational needs of the ward and theatre. This is a very skilled role and the situation could have ended in many different ways, which may have resulted in Jenny's needs and priorities not being central to decisions made.

In other situations, individuals' priorities cannot always be predicted and therefore need to be discussed. For example, people with long-term conditions are living longer, and children with life-limiting illnesses are surviving into adulthood. It is crucial, therefore, to 'remember that their priorities in life are likely to be different from those of healthcare professionals. Their personal stories tell of an alternative approach to living with chronic illness in which decisions are carefully considered within the life context of individuals' (Badlan 2006, p. 269).

In some countries, individuals can make different decisions about how the resources for their care are spent. This involves them knowing what services are available and how to access them. It can be wrongly assumed that everyone genuinely wants to self-care, when some individuals might not have the confidence or the motivation to do so. In addition, the priorities of the person with a disability or long-term condition might not be the same as that of their carers. When their friend or relative is away from the home, a carer might need that short space to have some precious time for themselves. If this does not happen, the whole care support system might fall apart. Therefore, priorities need to be carefully managed to ensure that all needs are met as far as possible, while still staying within the prearranged budget. The person with the disability or long-term condition might not be able to indicate what their choice would be, and in these cases a nurse might need to act as an advocate. This will be discussed further in Chapter 7.

Annells and Koch (2001) support the New Zealand study of Carter, *et al.* (2004), which states how important it is to accept people's priorities that are based on their feelings, values, norms and beliefs, because this is essential in ensuring that patient choice is central to decision making. This could be crucial to end-of-life decisions where, for example, a patient wants to prioritise dying at home, which might not fit with their daughter's priority of trying to keep the home situation as normal as possible for her children, as they are about to lose a close family member. Again, great skill is needed on the nurse's part to ensure that a compromise can be reached where all feel comfortable with the decision.

Therefore, it is important to work in partnership with individuals and communities so they can feel able to express their choices and priorities. However, it is also important not to raise expectations about what is possible to a point where people expect and demand services that cannot be provided within the resources available. Access to health information can be unreliable and misleading and patients' knowledge, competence, desires and limitations need to be respected. Staines (2008) says that patients can demand inappropriate treatments and products and can become angry and offensive when they are making their demands. Individual views should be respected, but this must be a two-way process as people need to realise that finances are finite, and also that opinions they have read might not be evidence-based and might not be appropriate for them or their condition.

As nurses, we need not only to seek ways of finding out what patients actually want or need, but also to balance these needs with what can realistically be provided within the healthcare systems in which we practise.

THOUGHTS FOR YOUR PRACTICE

- Think of a time when your organisational priorities have wrongly taken precedence over a patient's priorities.
- Do you think that on reflection there could have been better ways to take both sets of priorities into consideration?
- Do you feel that sometimes patients have unrealistic ideas about services or care that could be provided?
- If so, how do you try to address this?
- How do you increase someone's ability to make informed decisions about their health?
- How to you attempt to work with patients and their carers to try to resolve differences in their priorities and needs?

SUMMARY – LINKS TO COMPASSION AND CARING

In continuing our discussions of what compassionate care means in nursing practice, in this chapter we have focused on further aspects of person-centred care. This discussion has centred on the concepts of **choice** and **priorities**. Choice is important because it gives people power when they are in situations where they feel disempowered. Prioritisation is necessary in a resource constrained healthcare system where money needs to be spread as equitably as possible, bearing in mind the diversity of health needs to be met.

As nurses, we need to work in partnership with people to ensure that, as far as possible, these choices are real and not rhetoric and that people have as much information as they need to make informed decisions. This means that we need to change the power relationships so that we can work in concordance with people in our care. Nurses need to base their discussions on ethical principles, where they genuinely respect the beliefs and values of others, rather than assuming that everyone has the same priorities in life that they do.

REFERENCES

Annells M, Koch T. 'The real stuff': implications for nursing of assessing and measuring a terminally ill person's quality of life. *J Clin Nurs.* 2001; **10**(6): 806–12.

Badlan K. Young people living with cystic fibrosis: an insight into their subjective experience. *Health Soc Care Comm.* 2006; **14**(3): 264–70.

Bowling A, Gabriel Z. Lay theories of quality of life in older age. *Ageing Soc.* 2007; **27**(6): 827–48.

British Medical Association. *Decisions Relating to Cardiopulmonary Resuscitation: model information leaflet.* London: British Medical Association; 2002.

Carter H, MacLeod R, Brander P, *et al.* Living with a terminal illness: patients' priorities. *J Adv Nurs.* 2004; **45**(6): 611–20.

Coulter A. *Trends in Patients' Experience of the NHS.* Oxford: Picker Institute; 2006.

Cuff D. Sharing in partnership. In: Burley S, Mitchell E, Melling K, *et al.*, editors. *Contemporary Community Nursing.* London: Arnold; 1997.

Department of Health. *High Quality Care for All: NHS next stage review final report.* Cm 7432. London: Department of Health; 2008.

Gullick J, Shimadry B. Using patient and carer stories to improve quality of care. *Nurs Times.* 2008; **104**(10): 33–4.

Haggerty J, Reid R, Freeman G, *et al.* Continuity of care: a multidisciplinary review. *BMJ.* 2003; **327**(7425): 1219–21.

Hauge S, Heggen K. The nursing home as a home: a field study of residents' daily life in the common living rooms. *J Clin Nurs.* 2008; **17**(4): 460–7.

Hornby S, Atkins J. *Collaborative Care.* Oxford: Blackwell Science; 2000.

Koch T, Jenkin P, Kralik D. Chronic illness: self management: locating the 'self'. *J Adv Nurs.* 2004; **48**(5): 484–92.

Papadopoulos I, Lees S. Developing culturally competent researchers. *J Adv Nurs*. 2002; **37**(3): 258–64.

Staines R. Is patient power good for nurses? *Nurs Times*. 2008; **104**(13): 13–16.

Wallis N. My lifelong desire. *The Guardian*. 15 January 2007.

Wilkinson C. *Professional Perspectives in Health Care*. Basingstoke: Palgrave MacMillan; 2007.

Yu-Ching T, Ruey-Hsia W, Shu-Hui R. Relationship between perceived empowerment care and quality of life among elderly residents within nursing homes in Taiwan: a questionnaire survey. *Int J Nurs Stud*. 2006; **43**(6): 673–80.

CHAPTER 7

Empowerment and advocacy

Overview of the chapter

Key theme one – empowerment

- Case study
- Discussion
- How do we build therapeutic empowering relationships with patients and clients?
- Case study
- Discussion
- Thoughts for your practice
- How do nurses ensure that empowerment is a central focus in all patient contacts?
- Case study
- Discussion
- Thoughts for your practice

Key theme two – advocacy

- Case study
- Discussion
- Do we understand the true meaning of patient or client advocacy?
- Case study
- Discussion
- Thoughts for your practice
- How can we encourage patients and clients to be effective self-advocates?
- Case study
- Discussion
- Thoughts for your practice
- Summary – links to compassion and caring
- References

OVERVIEW OF THE CHAPTER

Throughout the previous chapters we have discussed different elements of compassionate care. We believe that encouraging empowerment in patients and clients is central to individualised patient-centred care. People do not always have the skills or confidence to express what they need or want in relation to their care. Nurses have a key role in helping them to develop these skills in order that they can become active participants, and not merely passive recipients of care.

Empowerment is a complicated concept and nurses need to develop their own skills in relation to empowering others. Sometimes acting as an advocate is an important part of the nursing role, because a patient or client is unable to act as an advocate for themselves. However, we need to be aware that while this might help their needs to be met at the time, this approach can be disempowering if it continues to be part of their ongoing care. People need to feel that their opinions are important, and that their voice is heard so that they feel more able to work in partnership with the professionals caring for them. This enables them to move from empowerment, through self-advocacy to become true self-determinants of their care.

KEY THEME ONE – EMPOWERMENT

CASE STUDY 7.1

Jack did not like hospitals; in fact, he had never been in one before. He knew it was unusual for someone in his early seventies not to have been in hospital before now, but he had been lucky and healthy all through his life.

The angina and shortness of breath had been a real shock to him, and the fact that he needed to have cardiac surgery was an even greater shock that he had dealt with in his usual way – by denying it was going to happen.

However, now that he was in hospital, denial was no longer an option. He had been admitted to the ward and could see other patients at various points in their recovery. He knew that he was anxious and afraid, but throughout his years in the armed forces these were emotions that he had been trained never to show. Therefore, he knew that he looked calm and in control, but that was a long way from how he was actually feeling.

A young nurse approached his bed and said that she wanted to talk to him about his operation the following day. He felt himself tense, but he managed to smile at her. She then started to explain, in what felt to him as the minutest of detail, what would happen during the operation, what tubes and intravenous infusions he would have and what would happen afterwards. He could feel his anxiety growing; he really did not want to know all this. It was bad enough to know that he was having the operation, without knowing exactly how vulnerable he was going to be at the time and afterwards. He knew that he coped much better without knowing things in advance, and although he knew that others might find this information reassuring, he certainly did not.

Discussion

It is often believed that people deal with situations better if they are prepared for them in advance. Therefore, giving detailed information about what will happen during and after an operation is usually considered to be good practice. However, the assumption that every individual will find this helpful and less threatening is just that: an assumption. Everybody deals differently with stressful situations, and while knowledge and information helps some people feel more in control of their circumstances, for others this information is threatening and disempowering. Nurses need to use all their skills to ensure that they are basing these types of discussion on the actual individual, rather than blindly following a protocol of good practice that dictates that people should be given certain information. However, these conversations are often a result, nowadays, of concerns about litigation. A patient could perhaps take legal action if they were not told about the consequence of an operation or medication in advance. Therefore, practitioners can feel that it is better to give all relevant information to a patient, despite the fact that the patient does not actually want to know the minutiae of every part of their care. This is a difficult balance and nurses obviously have to ensure that no crucial information is omitted, and that they are not at risk professionally. However, the concept of knowledge being empowering is not the case in Jack's situation. He is becoming more anxious with each new bit of information about his stay in hospital. Far from making him feel more in control, it is actually having the opposite effect. The nurse involved is unwittingly being disempowering.

So how do nurses know what is empowering and what is disempowering to people in their care? Wilkinson (2007) says that 'empowerment is a difficult concept to define and is sometimes easier understood by its absence as sensed in powerlessness, hopelessness, helplessness and alienation' (p. 31). This is an important point because it is often when things are disempowering that we think about empowerment at all. However, we need to recognise what empowerment actually is in order to develop the skills to act as agents of empowerment in our practice. Some people feel that the mere fact of passing on power is disempowering in itself, because it implies that we have more power in the first place. However, it is inevitably true that we are more comfortable in our workplaces than our patients usually are. We know the surroundings better, we know what resources are available and know from experience what patients or clients might find difficult in relation to their care. We want to reduce anxiety by passing on our knowledge, but this might not be helpful to some individuals.

Gibson (1991) discusses empowerment in terms of helping people to feel in control of their lives. This can involve assisting people to meet their own needs and solve their own problems by helping them to make the best use of available resources. In addition, Israel, *et al.* (1994) see empowerment as **individual** empowerment, **community** empowerment and **organisational** empowerment. For people to feel empowered as individuals they need to have a positive self-image and have a sense of being able to change things and to be effective. They also need to feel that they have some control over their own lives and can participate and influence decisions within the institutions with which they are involved. **Community** empowerment is seen as taking place when individuals and local organisations work together in using their joint knowledge and skills to meet the needs of their community. Examples of this will be seen and discussed further in this chapter. Israel (1994) perceives **organisational** empowerment as involving organisations empowering their own members and by sharing power democratically, which in turn influences and empowers the larger community.

It could be that nurses do not feel empowered themselves within their own organisations, in which case it can be difficult for them, in turn, to empower others. Therefore, the culture of any healthcare organisation should be based on a philosophy of organisational empowerment.

We intend, now, to take this further by discussing how we can build empowering relationships and how we ensure that empowerment is central to our practice.

How do we build therapeutic empowering relationships with patients and clients?

CASE STUDY 7.2

Rosie was absolutely petrified. She had found the lump in her breast last week and had gone to her doctor that day. Immediately, a referral had been made to her local breast care unit and here she was, early the following week, at the unit waiting for the results of various tests and scans she had this morning. Her husband, Tim, was sitting there at her side, and she could tell that he was terrified too. They had two young children, and breast cancer at 39 years of age was a terrible thought.

She had been introduced to Mr Shah, the breast care consultant, that morning and to Lorraine, the breast care nurse, and as they called her into the consulting room she found herself scanning their faces for any sign of what she was going to be told. As she and Tim sat down, Mr Shah immediately began to speak. He seemed to know that exchanging pleasantries at this point would have added to her distress. She heard him saying that, unfortunately, the lump was malignant and that she had breast cancer. At the word 'cancer' her panic was so severe that she could not seem to take in anything that he was saying after this. Again, both he and Lorraine seemed to know this and they moved their chairs closer and as Tim clutched frantically for one hand, Lorraine calmly held her other one. She searched their eyes again and immediately saw true kindness and understanding there. She felt herself relax enough to focus on what Mr Shah was saying. She felt that she could trust them. They seemed to understand how she was feeling and she did not doubt their knowledge and expertise.

Mr Shah told her that the lump was fairly small and there were no signs that the malignancy had spread to the lymph system. He then went on to discuss the different options available: surgery, chemotherapy and radiotherapy. These were words she had heard, of course, but she had never thought of them regarding herself. She suddenly realised that Mr Shah was asking her what she wanted in terms of treatment. How could she possibly know what was best? She felt her panic levels rising again. All she wanted was to have the best chance of full recovery if possible, or to live to see her children grow up or at least to get a bit older. She could hear herself bargaining in her mind: 'If I could just live until Naomi is 10 or until Jake is 18.' She found herself being distracted again and would have been totally unable to make the simplest decision, let alone contribute to a decision on her life or (potentially) death. She felt incapable of speech and she heard Tim say to Mr Shah in a broken voice that she had never heard before, 'What do you think is best?' She felt a sense of relief – of course, that is what they wanted to know. Mr Shah and Lorraine had years of experience and they must know what treatments gave her the best chance of survival. She wanted no part in this decision; she just wanted to follow their advice. She started to feel a little calmer as Mr Shah outlined what he would advise in terms of her specific tumour and her age, and Lorraine joined in with the effect this would have on her. She started to feel that there was a chance there could be a positive outcome in the end, as long as she followed their advice.

Discussion

Rosie was in a situation where she would naturally have felt disempowered. She was severely traumatised by this devastating diagnosis and was in uncharted territory and unfamiliar surroundings. It would have felt natural for the power to lie with the healthcare professionals, who had knowledge about breast cancer, generally, and her case specifically.

Millard (2006) discusses how the power base between healthcare professionals and patients or clients has to change. Relationships need to be more partnership orientated with shared decision making and, therefore, interpersonal interaction has to be central. Real involvement of the patient has to take place and the individuality of the person has to be taken into account. Rosie did not want to be an active participant in her care at this stage. She was still reeling from the diagnosis, which she had just been given. At a later stage she would have wanted to be involved in decisions about her care, but at the moment she just wanted to benefit from the expertise of specialists in the area of breast cancer. It would seem reasonable that the more serious someone's health issues are, the more likely this would be the case.

However, there are also people who never want to be active participants in their care, choosing instead to retain the traditional passive patient role. For example, older people have been brought up to respect the views of doctors, and women might not feel able to express their views to a male practitioner, particularly if they belong to an ethnic group where male supremacy is respected as the norm. This can be a deliberate choice and it can be very difficult to find out what the person actually wants when healthcare choices need to be made. Empowerment can be impossible to achieve in these circumstances, but as the nature of society changes, so do interactions between healthcare practitioners and patients. Sometimes this involves using other forms of communication, such as text messages and e-mails, which can empower people to become more involved in communication (Dean 2008). For example, children, young people and perhaps those at risk of forced marriage or domestic abuse, could feel safer and more comfortable using these forms of communication. Young people, particularly, tend to be able to divulge deeper feelings when they are not making eye contact or are unable to see the person they are communicating with. As communication networks change and people become more used to them, it could be easy to see how older housebound people could feel less isolated by communicating with nurses in this way.

The relationship is central to identifying what role the patient wants to play, so assessing this is essential. Mr Shah and Lorraine were very skilled in knowing that prolonged introductions at the start of the discussion would be inappropriate for Rosie and Tim in their highly stressed states. They also sensed that Rosie's anxiety was getting in the way of her being able to comprehend what she was being told. Additionally, they responded immediately to Tim's request for advice about what to do. However, this situation had to be assessed on an individual basis and although they had communicated bad news to many women in the past, no two conversations would have been exactly the same. As nurses, we need to vary our practice from patient to patient and not act in a uniform manner. This is because the extent to which a person feels empowered is strongly influenced by the attitude and behaviour of the nurse.

We need to remember that words are able to empower or disempower, put someone down or spur them on, confuse them or help them to understand, push someone away or draw them closer and build or destroy relationships. Therefore, we need to use our words and our interpersonal skills to aid our relationships with people in order for our interactions to be therapeutic.

In terms of nursing, a therapeutic relationship is a professional relationship that focuses on the patient or client and is centred on them and their needs. Professional boundaries need to be maintained and needs and goals need to be mutually identified with clear understanding and identification of roles. The nurse uses their expert communication skills in order to ensure that the person's needs are met in a way 'that is most appropriate for the patient and family' (Chilton, *et al.* 2004, p. 41).

A therapeutic relationship is an empowering one in which patient autonomy and self-determination are promoted, and the patient moves towards independence. Therefore, interactions are sensitive and based on patient choice and autonomy. Mr Shah and Lorraine were clearly trying to offer choices to Rosie, and they respected her autonomy and her right to make her own choices in life. However, Rosie was in an extremely serious and traumatic situation and her life chances were dependent on making the right decisions at this time. The healthcare professionals had more knowledge and experience than she did; they were not traumatised in the way she was and they could offer expert and objective advice. Having given her the option to make decisions for herself, based on their explanations of available treatments, they then sensitively responded to her need for guidance in the decision-making process.

Mr Shah and Lorraine clearly demonstrated therapeutic practice in this case study. Heron (1990, cited in Rungapadiachy 1999) identifies various supportive interventions based on the concept of care and love as a therapeutic tool for helping patients and clients. These include:

➤ expressing the loving feeling;
➤ expressing care;
➤ expressing concern;
➤ validating the client's worth;
➤ appropriate use of touch;
➤ sharing and self-disclosing (appropriately);
➤ giving free attention;
➤ encouraging the client;
➤ giving the client unconditional positive regard;
➤ accepting the client unconditionally;
➤ showing warmth.

The care, compassion and concern Mr Shah and Lorraine felt for Rosie was clearly demonstrated in their exclusive focus on her and Tim, which enabled Rosie to trust them. They altered their approach in response to her reactions and feelings and she felt respected and valued by them and was aware of their concern and sensitivity towards her. This is the essence of a therapeutic and empowering relationship.

THOUGHTS FOR YOUR PRACTICE

● How do you empower your patients and clients in order that they can become active participants in their care?
● Can you think of an example when you felt disempowered when you were a patient?
● What was it that made you feel that way?

- Can you think of a time when a patient or client might have felt disempowered by the care they received?
- How could this have been a more empowering experience for them?
- How can you build relationships that are as empowering as possible?
- How can you try to shift the power base in your relationships so that your patients feel more in control?
- How do you adapt your practice to meet the individual needs of your patients or clients?
- Can you think of ways in which your therapeutic relationships with patients could be enhanced in any way?
- How can you share all this knowledge with your colleagues and students in order to enhance the practice in your work environment?

How do nurses ensure that empowerment is a central focus in all patient contacts?

CASE STUDY 7.3

Andy was not looking forward to this visit. As a Community Children's Nurse, he spent much of his time involved in very sad situations where children were not going to recover. Parents were under immense pressure just dealing with their child's day-to-day needs, but the shadow of impending death was an ever-present reality. He always felt that it was a privilege to be accepted into the home when children were very ill or dying and to be there to help meet the child's needs as well as be a support to the family. However, he always felt the visit following a child's death particularly difficult. There was no child to focus on, no physical care to be given, and nothing to relieve the relentless grief of the parents. Parents really seemed to appreciate these visits, but it was always very difficult for the nurse involved, because they had usually known the child and their family for some time.

He took a deep breath and knocked on the door. Rosh answered the door, looking like he had not slept for a week, which was probably very nearly true. He welcomed him in with a smile that did not quite reach his eyes. As Andy went into the living area he saw Bel lying curled into a ball on the sofa. She sat up when she saw him, but it seemed to take every bit of energy she had left.

Anna had been the light of their lives and when she had contracted meningitis at the age of 18 months it seemed as if all life had gone out of their lives and they had continued to merely exist. Anna recovered to the extent that she could go home, but she was severely brain damaged and very weak. Rosh and Bel had nursed her with the help of the community nursing team and various other agencies for two more years. They had wanted as little help as possible, though, except during the day when they both worked; Anna was cared for by her paternal grandmother then. When it became clear in the last 10 days of her life that Anna could not survive much longer, Andy had had long discussions with Rosh and Bel, and with Rosh's mother, to ensure that they were as prepared as possible for her death.

Now that Anna had died he could feel that there was no focus to their lives. Bel had been a successful marketing manager and had continued to work up until the last few weeks of Anna's life. Rosh also has a busy job as a graphic designer and he too had worked until Anna's health had deteriorated further. Now, three weeks later, neither of them looked as if there was any immediate prospect of them going back to work, going out for an evening, seeing friends or doing anything more than merely existing.

Andy gently asked whether they were managing to sleep and eat adequately and Bel replied that she felt that it was a betrayal of their daughter for them to carry on living while she was not able to. They were eating rarely and minimally and they did not feel able to go to bed, they just fell asleep in the living room when the exhaustion got too much. Andy continued to ask questions about their lives after Anna had died and became more and more concerned with what he was hearing. They were not visiting anyone or allowing anyone to visit, including Rosh's mother. Andy said that they would never forget Anna or stop mourning her loss. However, they would gradually return to their previous activities and would even start to enjoy them, or become involved with new interests. Far from being a betrayal of Anna if they started to do normal things again, it was a tribute to her if their lives managed to become meaningful again. He said that they would know when it was right to start doing things again, but that small things, like sleeping in their own bed, were a start. Bel looked at him with a small amount of hope in her eyes and she turned to Rosh and said that it would be good to see his mother again, and the rest of his family. Rosh nodded and said that he knew that his mother was very distressed too, and was finding this apparent rejection of her very hard. He agreed that it was time to start reaching out to their families and friends again, who he knew were just waiting to receive a phone call to say that they wanted to see them.

Discussion

Bel and Rosh were obviously in severe distress and were not coping with life at all. Anna had meant the world to them; Andy knew this, but he also knew that the isolated way they were living at the moment was not helping in their bereavement. They needed to be able to access all the support that this popular couple had in their close circle of family and friends. However, he also did not want to appear critical of their current way of living or try to tell them what to do. Only they would know when they were ready to start doing normal activities again. Some people almost needed permission to start resuming life again and it needed a great deal of sensitivity on Andy's part to start to suggest this without appearing as if he did not understand the depth of their loss.

The study by Fazil, *et al.* (2004) on Pakistani and Bangladeshi families who have children with severe disabilities in the Birmingham area of the UK, highlights the importance of empowerment operating within the social, cultural and familial context of people's lives. This paper says that empowerment approaches that can make a real difference need to focus on three key areas.

1 Tackling those social processes and networks that would deny people the possibility of achieving their full potential.
2 Enabling the development of new social networks.
3 Nurturing those existing networks that do work.

Andy is clearly encouraging this in his discussion with Rosh and Bel. They have a good social network from which they are isolated at the moment. They might find that not all their relationships stand up to the strain that Anna's death might put on them. They also might find that new relationships and means of support become important to them, but at the moment they are denying themselves this possibility. This is a totally natural grief reaction, but there are not many people from whom they would accept this advice. Andy has been part of Anna's life and death and knows them well, so this puts him in a unique position to start making positive suggestions that might empower them to start to live their lives without Anna.

McCabe (2004) differentiates between authoritative interventions, which direct or control people's behaviour, and facilitative interventions, which empower people. McCabe stresses the importance of patient-centred communication in terms of 'communication that invites and encourages the patient to participate and negotiate in decision making regarding their own care' (p. 42). Andy was negotiating and feeling his way in this discussion and would have been encouraging Rosh and Bel to take an active part in the conversation. In a Taiwanese study, Tu, Wang and Yeh (2006) say that it is important to understand what constitutes quality of life in a particular culture in order to deliver empowered care, and, again, Andy was well aware of the family dynamics and the family and cultural norms.

Halldorsdottir (1997) suggests there are five modes of 'being with another'.

1 Empowering – which involves a sense of partnership where all parties speak and listen and contribute to the discussion.
2 Encouraging – where some power is shared in a supportive and reassuring manner.
3 Passive – where there is a lack of attentiveness or concern.
4 Discouraging – where there is insensitivity or indifference, which feels cold and dismissive.
5 Disempowering – which depersonalises and demands subordination and sometimes involves coercion or bullying.

These five modes can result in different feelings for the patient.
➤ Empowered – relieves the feeling of vulnerability; enables the patient to feel legitimate as a patient.
➤ Encouraged – gives a sense of security and comfort and the patient feels cared for and supported, but not empowered.
➤ Passive – where the patient feels alone, unsupported and uncared for.
➤ Discouraged – which limits the sense of freedom and diminishes the sense of control of the individual concerned.
➤ Disempowered – this causes severe distress and despair.

Andy is careful to be empowering by working in partnership with Rosh and Bel so that they do not feel that their grief reaction is abnormal. However, he is also encouraging by suggesting, in a sensitive and supportive manner, that they start to let people into their lives again in order to increase their level of support. It would have been much easier for him to just be supportive himself, and not challenge their social isolation. They might have felt comforted and reassured by his visit, but not empowered to move their lives forward.

As nurses, it can feel easier to give comfort rather than challenge or empower people because this takes more time at any given moment. However, this challenge often results in people becoming more independent which is much more positive and can involve less time overall. Unfortunately, there are many examples of times when nurses can be passive, cold and dismissive. In addition, particularly with people who are very vulnerable, nurses can be discouraging because it is quicker to do things for others, rather than giving them the time to do things for themselves. At the furthest end of the continuum, disempowering attitudes, which demand obedience and can be bullying, can cause a level of distress and despair that often stops an individual taking any initiative ever again. We need to challenge passive, discouraging and disempowering behaviour in others at all times, and take action so that this does not become common practice, or become embedded into the culture of the organisation or practice area.

Empowerment is crucial in nursing and there are times when we need to act as advocates for people in our care. However, it is important to understand the role of advocacy in leading to self-advocacy and hopefully self-determination. These challenging concepts will now be discussed in greater detail.

THOUGHTS FOR YOUR PRACTICE

- Think of a time when you tried to ensure that empowerment of an individual was the central focus of your care.
- What made this a positive experience for you and the patient or client?
- How has this experience influenced your current practice?
- What facilitative approaches do you use in your practice to ensure that your patients feel empowered?
- How do you ensure that your patients or clients benefit from culturally sensitive empowered care?
- Can you think of times when you have tried to reassure or comfort a patient, rather than gently challenging them to take more of a part in self-caring?
- How could you have turned this into a more empowering experience for the patient?

KEY THEME TWO – ADVOCACY

CASE STUDY 7.4

Real life patient experience

A woman with breast cancer in the UK campaigned successfully to be treated with a new cancer medication, which was not available on the National Health Service. Initially, she was refused this drug by her primary care trust (PCT). She was prepared to sell her house, but fortunately, following a high profile media campaign, she managed to raise £25000 in just two months, nearly enough to fund her own treatment. She says, 'Then I heard about a Human Rights Act case in the news where someone claimed that as a human being they had a right to life, so I went to a top human rights solicitor with the same argument and he said I might have a case. Her Member of Parliament then called for a debate in the House of Commons on the issue.

Shortly afterwards, having reviewed her circumstances, her local PCT agreed to fund her treatment. She said, 'I'm a nurse and I believe in saving lives. There are so many women out there who are struggling to get this drug, and I won't stop campaigning until everyone, whoever they are, wherever they live, can get this drug based on their clinical need.'

After starting her treatment, she decided to put the money she no longer needed to good use. 'I used it to help other women all over the country get started on the drug, which is great! Instead of one life being saved, I've helped about twelve now!' (Web Site on Breast Cancer Care, ID 3286)

Discussion

The woman in this real life case was fighting for her life, but she felt empowered not only to fight for her own right to live, but also to be an advocate for others in her position. This was at the same time as suffering from the side effects of chemotherapy and caring for a son with a life-limiting illness. Most people in her situation would have been totally focused on their own survival. They would have had no emotional or physical capacity to care about the fate of others. She felt that everybody had an equal right to life, and that merely being successful in her fight for her own health was not enough. She is an inspiration to us all and a clear example of an advocate, not only for herself, but also for others.

Teasdale (1998) says that 'advocacy is about power. It means influencing those who have power on behalf of those who do not' (p. 1), and goes on to say that advocacy involves pleading, interceding or speaking for another.

> In other words, advocacy is required when people feel vulnerable and powerless. It is sad, but true that those who suffer from illness or disabilities frequently report precisely these feelings of vulnerability and powerlessness in their own dealings with members of the caring professions (Teasdale 1998, p. 1).

Bateman (2001) agrees with this and says 'there are many successful advocates who readily admit that they make poor self advocates' (p. 17). The woman in this real life story was able to be a successful advocate for others as well as a successful self-advocate, which is an unusual combination.

Kim-Godwin, Clarke and Barton (2001) say that advocacy is an important cultural skill and that 'advocacy involves not only recognising racism and ethnocentrism, but also doing something about it on behalf of clients and society' (p. 922). As nurses, how often have we seen someone being treated unfairly in terms of equity of healthcare provision, or because they are of a different social class, gender or ethnic group? When we see unfairness and disadvantage, empowerment is important and sometimes, in the short term, we might need to be strong advocates on patients' or clients' behalf. Then we can work towards empowering them sufficiently for them to become their own self-advocates.

In the following section we will discuss whether we understand what advocacy actually means and how we can try to encourage people to be effective self-advocates.

Do we understand the true meaning of patient or client advocacy?

CASE STUDY 7.5

Sylvia was sitting shaking on the sofa when Pauline arrived to dress her leg ulcer. Pauline could sense the tension in the air as soon as she walked in, as she usually could when she visited. Donna, Sylvia's daughter, was looking sulky and irritable, and Jason, her partner, would not make eye contact with her, but was looming over Sylvia in a way that must be making her feel very threatened. As soon as Pauline put her bag down, they said they were going out and did not know when they would be getting back. Pauline was concerned because Sylvia was unable to move on her own. It was coming up to lunchtime and she could not see any food prepared for Sylvia.

As soon as the door closed behind Donna and Jason, Sylvia seemed to relax her shoulders and breathe more regularly. Pauline waited for her to relax a little more and was just finishing dressing her wound when she casually asked how things were now that Donna's partner had moved in. Sylvia started to shake at the mention of Jason's name and as Pauline looked up she saw tears streaming down Sylvia's face. Closing her bag, Pauline went to sit on the sofa next to Sylvia. She knew that the relationship between Sylvia and Donna had been stormy for some time. Donna had come to live with her mother when her marriage split up and Pauline had often heard her shouting at Sylvia when she walked down the path. Pauline felt uneasy with Jason around. She did not really know why, but she sensed hostility whenever he was there. Donna seemed a little too eager to please him and there was never any interaction between him and Sylvia.

Pauline asked gentle probing questions and it was immediately clear that Sylvia was frightened of him. He would come into her room at night, when he got back from the pub, and shout and swear at her and put his face up very close to hers as he did so. He kicked the bed and shouted some more and then went out, leaving the door open. Sometimes he would return for more of the same and sometimes he did not; Sylvia never knew what was going to happen next. Donna also shouted at her and ridiculed her about her age, her infirmity, her leg ulcers – anything really. Sylvia never knew when she was going to get something to eat or drink, even though it was her pension that paid for the food in the first place.

Pauline was extremely alarmed by what she heard as it was much worse than she had suspected. She asked Sylvia what she wanted most and her immediate reply was that she wanted to get away from here. She could not face another night here, even though it was her own home. Sylvia immediately phoned the emergency care manager at social services and stressed the need for an urgent visit with a view to immediate re-housing. Pauline was explaining to Sylvia what would probably happen as a result of her phone call when she heard a car outside. Fearing it was Donna and Jason, she looked out of the window and saw to her relief that John, the care manager, was walking up the path instead. John pulled up a chair so that he was facing Sylvia and gently asked her to repeat what she had been telling Pauline. Pauline saw a brief look of anger in John's eyes as he looked away quickly; she knew that he could not bear to hear of abuse of older people. He turned back to Sylvia, smiled at her and said in a reassuring voice, 'Well, we need to get you out of here this afternoon, don't we?' Sylvia looked at him with such gratitude and John started to make some phone calls.

Discussion

Sylvia is very vulnerable in this situation. The risk of physical abuse from Jason is very high and the situation is escalating. Both Donna and Jason are being psychologically abusive in terms of being verbally abusive, swearing, bullying, blaming and humiliating Sylvia (Community and District Nursing Association 2003). They could be withholding food and fluids at times and probably ignore her most of the time when they are not humiliating or threatening her. She is not being treated with respect or dignity and she is being offered no choices in decisions that affect her life. She is probably just forced to be grateful when she is given any food, and probably has no choice over programmes to watch on television or when she sleeps. This is a gross invasion of her human rights.

Pauline and John work together to provide a safe environment for her as this is clearly an urgent situation. They act as advocates because empowerment is not an option in this situation. If Sylvia complained about Jason's behaviour, or argued back, her situation would probably get worse. For Sylvia, being taken away from her home could be a deeply disempowering experience, if she had not been involved in the decision making and was not so relieved at the proposed outcome. Sylvia did not feel in a position to stand up for herself. It had taken all her courage to tell Pauline what had been going on. Therefore, she needed Pauline and John to act as advocates and intercede on her behalf. Everyone should feel able to ask for help at times, and someone acting as an advocate is sometimes the only way for change to take place.

There is a continuum from empowerment to disempowerment. At the disempowerment end of the continuum, individuals, groups and communities may need external advocates. The intention should be that external advocacy is short term and that empowerment will return with help from skilled individuals. As Teasdale (1998) says 'external advocacy is necessary when clients have either exhausted the avenues open to them or when they are no longer in any fit state to plead their own case' (p. 73). Therefore, the intention is that people move from advocacy to empowerment and then self-advocacy. If this does not happen, then advocacy can make individuals and communities feel more disempowered, compounding their low self-worth and self-esteem (Hart and Freeman 2005). Inequalities in health can be perpetuated as a result, and nurses need to be aware that acting as advocates can be damaging to a person's or community's ability to function or solve problems for themselves.

THOUGHTS FOR YOUR PRACTICE

- Think of an example from your practice where you have acted as an advocate for a patient or client.
- Was this a positive experience? If so, what happened as a result?
- If not, what do you feel could have been a more positive outcome?
- Have you ever acted as an advocate for a group of patients or clients or a local community?
- Could you see yourself in this role in the future? If yes, how could you see this taking place?
- Have there been situations in your practice where you have called on additional external advocates to support your patient or client?
- If so, was this appropriate, and why?
- If this was inappropriate, why was this the case and how could this situation have had a more positive outcome?
- How did this form of advocacy help to empower your client or patient?

How can we encourage patients and clients to be effective self-advocates?

CASE STUDY 7.6

June seemed to have lived in fear all her life and had always lived in the same area of supported housing. This area of high rise and multi-level accommodation had many dark alleyways and corners and, after dark, it took on an even more menacing feel. It became the territory of gangs, who were in conflict with each other, drug dealers, and pimps and the working women who were controlled by them. Only the young people, who had the bravado and attitude to feel that this was also their territory, had felt safe to venture out at these times. However, they took knives and other means of protection with them and they raced their cars down the narrow streets.

June had children of her own and she felt frightened for them. She could never relax while they were out and constantly felt that one night they might never come back at all. Knife crime was rife and several young people had died from stab wounds in the area. However, although she was only too aware of the risks of living in this neighbourhood, she felt a sense of pride in her local community. They would always help each other out and there were many parents who wanted to bring about change for the future. She felt that people who lived there deserved more out of life and better futures, but they needed to have opportunities to make this happen.

This is why she had set up a group of like-minded people to try to make a difference. As nobody wanted to move into the area, there was an empty flat that the authorities had agreed they could use for communal purposes. This flat was now the hub of many different activities in the day, and in the evenings too.

There was a large kitchen and this was used to provide breakfast for children whose parents were unable to prepare food for them in the mornings; for example, shift workers on nights or who worked early shifts and young parents without the desire or domestic skills to make breakfast for their children. June was aware that having breakfast was important in helping children to concentrate and achieve more at school. During the day, the flat was also used to help people to cook on limited budgets and, for those new to this country, to learn how to cook with ingredients that were available locally. It also had computers and there was help available for people to build up their literacy and computer skills and to write application forms that might help them to get work, which they had never been able to apply for before. Also, there were sessions on budgeting, safety and raising self-esteem, as well as beauty sessions and opportunities for people to meet as a group if they had similar interests. Also, older people who had not felt able to come out of their flats were starting to meet and start up different activities. After school, children would come back again. They were always hungry and food was available. They were given priority for using the computers for their homework, which they had never bothered to do before.

In the evening, there were enough people around to travel to and from the flat together and any suggestions for things to do were taken seriously by all involved. At the moment, there was a strong movement for parents to stop their children going out with knives. They had also been very successful in working with the police and other agencies to reduce drug dealing and set up traffic calming measures to prevent the joyriding that had always happened in the area.

The flat had been running for two years now and June could see the sense of ownership and community that was starting to take place as a result. Self-esteem was much higher in the young people. They were starting to leave school with better qualifications and job prospects were increasing within the community. Young people were starting to use the flat too, which allowed them to access health advice about smoking, substance misuse and safe sex. June hoped that, eventually, better prospects, contraceptive advice and raised self-esteem would reduce the high number of teenage pregnancies in the area. People who were new to the country were being accepted into the community more and there was much more shared learning and socialising taking place. She believed strongly that knife crime would be reduced dramatically if all parents worked together on this. Overall, she was delighted with how things had developed since this initiative had been started.

Discussion

It is very clear that June is an empowered person who has a sense of social responsibility and feels that she wants to make a difference in her own community. She is empowered to the point that she can be an advocate for both herself and others. She also has a sense of self-determination and self-efficacy that allows her to feel that she can take some control over her own destiny and can be effective in this initiative. Self-determination, respect of others as people in their own right, excellent communication and networking skills are key components of advocacy.

Nurses have a role in helping to raise self-esteem in their patients and clients, who can then feel more in control of their lives, their health and their lifestyle options. School nurses and health visitors can have a major influence in enhancing self-esteem and in giving advice about sexual, physical and emotional health to children, young people and their parents. In turn, these people can help others to develop themselves and maximise their opportunities in relation to quality of life.

In the Ottowa Charter (WHO 1986), empowerment is seen as helping people to gain control over their lives. This is perceived as both a prime goal in its own right as well as a major means of achieving equity. In order to achieve this goal, a supportive environment has to be created at all levels and this can be through building healthy public policy and by strengthening individuals' personal skills, abilities, confidence levels and capabilities.

Individuals, groups and communities need to feel that they have some control over their lives, as June clearly demonstrated. This involves some awareness of the 'root causes of their problems and a readiness to act on this awareness' (Wilkinson 2007, p. 34). Again, June and her friends clearly understand what is causing problems in their community and they are working on:

➤ building self-esteem in individuals and groups;
➤ encouraging a sense of community identity and of belonging within the local community;
➤ maximising chances of success, for example, by providing an environment where children and young people can study effectively and can get help with job applications;
➤ giving people life skills in terms of budgeting, cooking and keeping safe;
➤ giving advice on sexual health, drugs, substance misuse and other lifestyle and health advice;
➤ increasing communication within the community to reduce social isolation and a sense of social responsibility across age, gender and racial boundaries, for others who were struggling with life;
➤ increasing networks with health, social care and education agencies, as well as informal advice and support agencies.

Therefore, June and her friends were able to act as powerful self-advocates, which involves personal self-confidence and the ability to speak out on their own behalf, and the behalf of others, to bring about change. Teasdale (1998) says that 'empowerment means giving information or support to individuals to help them to undertake self-advocacy' (p. 51). Self-advocacy involves people feeling able to express their own needs. Nurses can encourage this by giving sufficient information to enable patients and clients to make informed choices. Patients and clients have to feel that they have genuinely got the capacity to make choices and bring about change and that they have a sense of autonomy. There is often a greater opportunity for patients and clients to exercise control in the community than in the hospital setting. Collective self-advocates, as demonstrated by June and her friends, can bring about change in the law and can change circumstances and the services available. Carers can act as external or self-advocates and patients and clients can act as self-advocates, but they often need support from nurses to do so. External advocacy should only be necessary when an individual, group or community feel disempowered. This should be short-lived and nurses should carefully assess the extent of disempowerment and the extent to which they need to act as agents of empowerment or advocacy in order to maximise the chances of self-advocacy and self-determination in their patients and clients.

THOUGHTS FOR YOUR PRACTICE

- Think of an example from your practice where you supported an individual patient or client to become a self-advocate.
- What did you do in this situation?
- Did this work well? If so, why?
- If this was not successful, why do you think this was the case?
- If you cannot think of a situation such as this in your practice so far, try to think of ways in which you can encourage self-advocacy in the future.
- How can you share this concept with colleagues and students?
- How can you help your patients and clients to become more autonomous individuals?
- Can you think of an example where you encouraged a group to take more control over their particular situation?
- If so, was this approach effective, and if so, why?
- If not, what do you think were the barriers to people taking greater control over their life circumstances?
- Can you think of ways that you could encourage group or community autonomy in your practice? If so, how would you share your ideas with colleagues and students?

SUMMARY – LINKS TO COMPASSION AND CARING

By focusing on the complex concepts of empowerment and advocacy, we hope that this chapter has challenged you to review what these mean for you and your practice.

Unless we are committed to building therapeutic relationships with patients and clients, which involve supporting people to take more control over their lives, our commitment to being compassionate in our caring could be questioned.

We have to realise that our healthcare environments are inherently paternalistic and disempowering. In addition to this, people feel vulnerable through their ill health, or challenges in life, and they may be in an unfamiliar environment. Nurses have to be very careful because patients' and clients' vulnerability can mean that their self-esteem and autonomy could be easily and severely compromised. We can be guilty of expecting people to 'fit in' to our care environment, which at times could be necessary, but at other times there could more flexible ways of helping people to feel more in control in a strange and depersonalising environment.

As nurses, we can feel very threatened by articulate, knowledgeable and assertive patients or clients, or by those who are unable to express their views in a less aggressive manner. We have to remember that people may be genuinely knowledgeable about their health condition, or they can feel frightened and out of control. It is our role to encourage people to feel comfortable in their care environment, or in their discussions with us. We need to let go of some of the power we have traditionally held and work in genuine partnership with our patients and clients in order that they can feel they have active choices concerning their care.

Not only can comfort can be used to empower, but also it can disempower people, and we need to ensure that we use this in a positive and short-term manner so that people can regain control over their lives as quickly as possible. We need to actively look for ways in which we can encourage people to be as autonomous as possible, as this does not tend to be a natural consequence of our care.

REFERENCES

Bateman N. *Advocacy Skills for Health and Social Care Professionals*. London: Jessica Kingsley Publishers; 2001.

Chilton S, Melling K, Drew D, *et al. Nursing in the Community*. London: Arnold; 2004.

Community and District Nursing Association. *Responding to Elder Abuse*. London: Community and District Nursing Association; 2003.

Dean A. Communicating with patients using email and the internet. *Nurs Times*. 2008; **104**(7): 29–30.

Fazil Q, Wallace L, Singh G, *et al.* Empowerment and advocacy: reflections on action research with Bangladeshi and Pakistani families who have children with severe disabilities. *Health Soc Care Comm*. 2004; **12**(5): 389–97.

Gibson C. A concept analysis of empowerment. *J Adv Nurs*. 1991; **16**: 354–61.

Halldorsdottir S. *Clinical Knowledge and Praxis in Nursing*. Philadelphia, PA: Sage; 1997.

Hart A, Freeman M. Health 'care' interventions: making health inequalities worse not better? *J Adv Nurs*. 2005; **49**(5): 502–12.

Heron J. Helping the client: a creative practical guide. In: Rungapadiachy D, editor. *Interpersonal Communication and Psychology for Healthcare Professionals*. Oxford: Butterworth Heinemann; 1999.

Israel B, Checkoway B, Schulz A, *et al.* Health education and community empowerment: conceptualising and measuring perception of individual, organisational and community control. *Health Educ Behav*. 1994; **21**(2): 149–70.

Kim-Godwin Y, Clarke P, Barton L. A model for the delivery of culturally competent community care. *J Adv Nurs*. 2001; **35**(6): 918–25.

McCabe C. Nurse-patient communication: an exploration of patients' experiences. *J Clin Nurs*. 2004; **13**(1): 41–9.

Millard L, Hallett C, Luker K. Nurse-patient interaction and decision-making in care: patient involvement in community nursing. *J Adv Nurs*. 2006; **55**(2): 142–50.

Teasdale K. *Advocacy in Healthcare*. Oxford: Blackwell Science; 1998.

Tu Y, Wang R, Yeh S. Relationship between perceived empowerment care and quality of life among elderly residents within nursing homes in Taiwan: a questionnaire survey. *Int J Nurs Stud*. 2006; **43**(6): 673–80.

Wilkinson C. *Professional Perspectives in Healthcare*. Basingstoke: Palgrave MacMillan; 2007.

World Health Organization. *Ottawa Charter for Health Promotion*. Copenhagen: World Health Organization; 1986.

www.breastcancercare.org.uk/content.php?page_id=3286

CHAPTER 8

Conclusion: Compassion in nursing – the way forward

Overview of the chapter

Key theme one – compassion

- Case study
- Discussion
- What are the challenges to compassionate care in nursing?
- Case study
- Discussion
- Thoughts for your practice
- How do nurses work towards overcoming these challenges in practice?
- Case study
- Discussion
- Thoughts for your practice

Key theme two – caring

- Case study
- Discussion
- How do we ensure that caring is central within our nursing practice?
- Case study
- Discussion
- Thoughts for your practice
- How can we continue to challenge a lack of caring in our own practice and that of others?
- Case study
- Discussion
- Thoughts for your practice
- Summary – links to compassion and caring
- References

OVERVIEW OF THE CHAPTER

We hope you have found that the previous chapters have helped you to identify ways to enhance your practice in relation to compassion and caring. In Chapter 1, we tried to identify what compassion and caring actually mean to patients and clients in terms of nursing care, and how nurses can build these important elements into their nursing practice to a greater extent. Different people have different perspectives on what compassion and caring actually are, and as we have said at various points in this book, it is often easier to see when a particular trait is missing, rather than to actually say what it is, or when it is evident in practice.

Having based the book on the different themes that we think are central to compassionate and caring practice, we now want to look at the potential challenges that prevent nurses being as compassionate as they would like to be. We will then discuss possible ways to work towards addressing these challenges. We need to ensure that caring is central to our nursing practice and we can only do this by challenging uncaring practice in ourselves and others. These points will be discussed more fully in this concluding chapter.

KEY THEME ONE – COMPASSION

CASE STUDY 8.1

Real life patient experience

I was admitted as an emergency to Aspen Ward at the Cumberland Infirmary two weeks ago and stayed in two nights, for what was to be a very emotional and traumatic time for me and my husband. All the staff on the ward that looked after me were amazing. They spent time with me, showed real compassion and patience and nothing was too much bother. They answered the nurse call quickly, even though I know they were busy with other things. I was not left in pain for long and I was treated with the utmost respect and dignity.

I needed to have surgery on the second day and again the anaesthetic staff and particularly the young anaesthetist and two recovery nurses who were assigned to me were wonderful. They were all so professional, but again, as on Aspen, they were compassionate at such a sad and difficult time for me. Their care for me was outstanding. (Web Site on Patient Opinion, ID 7846)

Discussion

The patient in this real life experience actually says that she was treated with compassion at a sad and difficult time. So exactly why did she feel that the care she received was compassionate? This case study highlights a positive approach to compassionate care. The themes within the chapters of this book that comprise compassionate care (*see* Table 8.1, column 1, on the following pages) have been used to identify some of the reasons why the patient felt this was the case (*see* Table 8.1, column 2). We have also used these themes to identify challenges to compassionate care that need to be taken seriously within our nursing practice (*see* Table 8.1, column 3).

This framework for compassionate practice covers many different aspects of compassionate care. In the real life patient experience described in Case study 8.1, the patient clearly believes that she has been treated with compassion, and several aspects of this framework appear to have been particularly important for her. Nurses were clearly empathetic, sensitive and responsive to her needs and she also felt she was treated with dignity and respect. However, the nurses involved in her care demonstrated less explicitly that they were listening to her and forming a therapeutic relationship, which is a fundamental part of empowerment. Cultural competence and diversity were not necessarily evident in this scenario. However, if nurses had not respected her as an individual, and had been judgemental, the patient would not have perceived this as compassionate care. In the same way, if nurses had not acted as advocates if necessary, or offered choice and focused on her priorities, then again she would not have perceived her care as being compassionate. In the patient's opinion, the compassion that she was shown by the nurses demonstrated their professionalism. It is important that nurses recognise the links between professionalism and compassion.

We will discuss the challenges to compassionate care (as highlighted in Table 8.1) in more depth in the following section, together with potential solutions for addressing these challenges.

TABLE 8.1 Framework for compassionate practice – evidence and challenges

Column 1	Column 2	Column 3
Theme	Evidence	Challenges
Empathy	• Patient seen as a person • Needs understood • Nurse engaged with patient • Communication skills reflect understanding • Genuineness • Non-judgemental attitude • Nurse emotionally intelligent – acting on their feelings and those of others	• Patients mirroring the negative mood of the nurse in terms of stress or distress • Poor communication is irreversible and causes uncertainty or distress • The nurse may want to distance themselves from others' distress • The nurse may have had recent experiences that make it difficult to show empathy
Sensitivity	• Nurse senses vulnerability • Nurse offers emotional comfort • Patient-centred care	• Time constraints • Poor use of humour • Emphasis on technology • Emphasis on science not art of nursing • Limited time to build relationships • Moral distress of not being able to provide compassionate care • Caring overload causing desensitisation
Dignity	• Patient treated with dignity • Patient treated as a person • Patient feels listened to • Patient feels understood • Prioritises what is important to the patient	• Culture of the ward or practice area does not promote dignity • Meeting targets seen as more important than dignity issues • Lack of leadership that promotes dignity • Inadequate staffing levels
Respect	• Patient treated with respect • Patient respected as a person • Confidentiality maintained • Trusting relationships developed	• People are stereotyped • Cultural norms and values not understood

TABLE 8.1 (*continued*)

Column 1 Theme	Column 2 Evidence	Column 3 Challenges
Listening	• Patient has time to talk • Nurse actively listens to the patient	• Nurse stress or anxiety • Offering false reassurance • Belittling patient experiences or concerns • Other behaviours that block communication
Responding	• Caring for and about the patient • Use of therapeutic touch	• Focus exclusively on nursing tasks
Diversity	• Differences seen as assets • Non-judgemental attitude • Inclusive care	• Nurse being too busy to adapt care to actual person • Judgemental attitude • Person treated like an outsider
Cultural competence	• Cultural sensitivity • Cultural awareness • Cultural skills • Cultural knowledge	• Misunderstanding of patient norms and values • Different interpretation of behaviour and concerns
Choice	• Patient given choice • Patient seen as a partner • Care based on concordance • Patient makes informed decisions	• Relationships with nurses enforced • Patient has no power and no choice • Privacy not maintained • Patient does not feel in control
Priorities	• Patient's needs prioritised • Continuity of care	• Patient forced to self-care • Fragmentation due to too many staff involved
Empowerment	• Helped to retain some control in an alien environment • Patient part of decision making • Therapeutic relationships	• Authoritative rather than facilitative approach • Too much comfort and too little challenge • Disempowering culture of practice area
Advocacy	• Empowering approach • Encourages self-determination • Minimising dependency	• Maximises dependency • Reduces confidence to take responsibility

What are the challenges to compassionate care in nursing?

CASE STUDY 8.2

Lisa – part 1

Lisa had been lying in the same position for some hours, just staring at the wall with her back to the others in her bay of four patients. She was only 18 and the patients in her bay frightened her. One poor woman was clearly close to death and was breathing in a very unnatural way, and the pauses between her breaths were getting longer and longer. She had never seen a dead person before and she really did not want to see one now, particularly when she was feeling so ill and vulnerable.

Another patient was moaning all the time and she had heard nurses try to calm her. She did not appear to be in pain – it seemed to be an almost involuntary response for her – but Lisa wondered if it was indicating deep distress, which she was unable to express.

The third patient was carrying out a conversation with herself, which did not appear to resolve any of the anxieties she clearly had. Lisa felt desperately sorry for these other women, but she could not help them, and the nurses were really just as powerless, although she could see that they cared.

Lisa really felt as if she did not belong here. She felt desperately lonely and far away from anyone who cared about her. She knew that her parents were on their way to visit her, but that would not help her after they were gone.

Nurses had been in to change her intravenous infusion bag regularly, but all they did was look at her name tag and then change the bag. She could not blame them because she could hear how busy they were. She heard approaching footsteps and waited for the same thing to happen again.

Discussion

Lisa was clearly very frightened and distressed by what was happening around her, and despite various nursing interventions where the nurses had carried out aspects of care, she was not feeling cared for or cared about. We believe that there are many challenges to compassionate care (identified in Table 8.1, column 3) and that these can be drawn together under three areas:

1   The attitude of the nurse.
2   The culture of the practice area.
3   Resourcing issues.

We will now discuss these three areas in this section in greater detail because a common assumption is that the reason nurses are unable to demonstrate their ability to be compassionate is largely because of a lack of adequate resourcing. While financial issues are an undeniable pressure, this can be seen as a reason to excuse nursing care that falls short of the levels of compassion that nurses and patients would both want to give and receive.

In the case study above, Lisa is not being treated in a compassionate manner. While the nurses are undoubtedly busy, the lack of compassion of individual nurses who fail to notice or engage with Lisa's distress is also a factor, as is the culture of the ward, which does not challenge this attitude and enables this approach to be replicated by different nurses involved in her care.

Firstly, **the attitude of the nurse** is essential in ensuring that there are no barriers to compassion on a personal or professional level. A nurse working in a particular area of practice can find the environment stressful and can therefore employ negative coping strategies to deal with this stress. Both inappropriate use of humour and poor communication can be irreversible from the patient's point of view. Other behaviours that block communication, such as avoiding eye contact, lack of active listening and not being genuine with patients and clients, will always have a negative impact on compassionate care. Nurses can inadvertently or purposefully belittle people in their care, they can be judgemental and stereotype people, or give false reassurance that neither they nor the patients actually believe.

As nurses, we might have personal reasons why we cannot demonstrate empathy towards a patient or client. Our behaviour might be due to personal experiences or beliefs, which at this point we cannot alter. We might feel that there are too many demands on our caring capacity and we could be experiencing caring overload. Therefore, we might need to distance ourselves from the patient in order to cope with our feelings, but this can lead to a form of 'moral distress', which can make us feel guilty and increase the levels of stress and distress on us personally. Patients and clients can sense this stress and distress and may mirror our behaviour, which makes interactions more difficult and can have a negative impact on patients' recovery or experience.

It is important for us to realise, as nurses, that true compassion involves being fully immersed in the condition of being human. Taken to its full conclusion, this means we would have to 'cry with those in misery, mourn with those who are lonely and weep with those in tears . . . being weak with the weak, vulnerable with the vulnerable and powerless with the powerless' (Nouwen, McNeill and Morrison 1982, cited in von Dietze and Orb 2000, p. 169). If this were true, we would not be able to be any help at all because, taken to its end point, this involves identifying completely with those in our care, to the detriment of being able to be objective and to problem solve.

In addition, we decided to be nurses in order to care for others, and this involves showing compassion. Goleman (2004) says that compassion is diametrically opposite to cruelty and anger. We might not actually be cruel or unkind, but when our standards slip below that which we would perceive as caring, this creates a stress of its own. If compassion is real and not contrived, this benefits us as nurses as well as the people in our care. This makes us feel more positive and can have a calming effect, which reduces our level of stress. Therefore, we need to be self-aware and recognise when our personal or professional stress starts to impact on our nursing care, and try to take steps to remedy this. We might also need to challenge the environment in which we work, which might be contributing to our stress because we cannot provide the care that we know is essential. We also need to recognise negative attitudes in others – the antithesis of compassion – and challenge these attitudes in a supportive and compassionate manner.

Secondly, **the culture of the practice area** is essential in enabling individual nurses to provide compassionate care. The care environment can limit or increase the caring capacity of individuals and the whole caring team. Patients can sometimes feel that they are being forced to care for themselves when they would rather have someone else caring for them. We need to understand this ourselves and convey it to patients, as sometimes they may want more care than we can provide, and in these situations self-caring may be the only option. However, there have to be limits to self-care and we need to be sure in our own minds where these limits lie. In addition, if we provide too much comfort and too little challenge to patients, we can inadvertently disempower them. They can feel that they are unable to do things for themselves, which increases their level of dependency. This is a delicate balance and we need to ensure that these decisions are made based on the patients' needs and not on how much time we have available to care for them. Rescheduling certain care to a different time in the day could allow us more time to build patients' confidence to self-care, rather than leaving them to their own devices, which can also be disempowering.

We need to understand that each patient or client is an individual that cannot and should not be stereotyped into what we believe a particular group of people want or need. Different people behave in different ways when they are unwell or under stress, and this could be influenced by their culture, age or gender, or it could be their own reaction to their situation. While we need to try to understand the norms and values of different groups of people, we must not make assumptions about what they might need. Patients and clients might find it hard to identify with particular nurses and yet there is often little choice about who carries out their care, particularly in a community environment. This needs to be handled sensitively so that compromises can be reached if possible.

As nurses, if we reduce nursing down to specific nursing tasks and place too great an emphasis on the science of nursing to the exclusion of the art of nursing, we lose the essence of what nursing should be about. In addition, if we are autocratic rather than facilitative in our interactions with patients and clients we again lose the compassionate centre of nursing practice. McCabe (2004) says that there can be an organisational culture that not only reinforces poor communication, but also encourages patients being approached for functional or task-orientated reasons alone. McCormack and McCance (2006) highlight the fact that the provision of physical care is often essential as a way in to providing person-centred care. They emphasise that qualified nurses need to remember this in the care they provide.

However, qualified nurses should be the leaders and innovators of nursing care, and therefore compassionate care. Nurses who are leaders and managers within their practice environment need to take this role seriously. They are responsible for the culture of the care environment and for ensuring that patients' privacy and dignity are promoted and upheld. They need to challenge poor or inadequate practice in a supportive and educational manner. Nurses can be bullied or intimidated into not challenging or reporting unacceptable practice that lacks dignity and compassion. They can feel at risk of being suspended for whistleblowing and fearful of being involved in industrial tribunals. Von Dietze and Orb (2000) say that a competitive environment means that nurses are in competition with each other rather than caring for each other. Unhealthy competition between nurses is not only detrimental to other nurses, but negatively affects the care they give. Therefore, team dynamics and a positive team environment are essential in being caring and supportive of others in the caring team, as well as the patients in our care. In a Norwegian study, Hem and Heggen (2004) say that there should be a collective ability and willingness to put compassion into practice: 'It is not enough that one nurse is aware and supportive of a patient in distress. It has to be a collective response' (p. 28).

Finally, **resourcing issues** and financial constrains undoubtedly place great pressures on nurses who are trying to provide quality nursing care. An Australian study carried out by von Dietze and Orb (2000) says that resources are a limiting factor that restricts the ability of nurses to allow time and resources for true compassionate care. In addition to this, reduced time in hospital and the resulting reduction in contact can have a detrimental effect on nurses' ability to build relationships with patients. This is also true within a community environment where nurses have less time to visit patients and clients, and there can be a lack of continuity in care due to increased skill mix, different agencies involved and the different roles that nurses have. Financial decisions are made in relation to different agencies' budgets and this can detract from the patient-focused approaches that epitomise compassionate care. Achieving pre-set targets defined by government policies can be seen as more of a priority than focusing attention on quality care for patients and clients. In another Australian study, Williams and Irurita (2004) say that changes to organisations (i.e. more technology, limited budgets and increased emphasis on direct outcomes) have led to a decrease in emphasis on psychosocial care 'as it is more abstract and difficult to measure than other outcomes relating to physical care' (p. 808). They say that time to devote to psychosocial care and emotional comfort is limited.

Financial pressures are a reality in healthcare with demographic shifts towards people living longer and with more complex health needs. The challenge to nurses is maintaining compassion as a central focus of their care within this financially driven environment. Nurses need to take a leadership role in ensuring that practice is as quality-driven and patient-focused as possible. Nurses also need to be taught how to stay motivated to nurse in busy practice environments with many different pressures and time constraints. If nursing care is to be considered caring then compassion has to remain a central focus for nurses.

THOUGHTS FOR YOUR PRACTICE

- What negative coping strategies do you use or have you seen in others, when you are working under pressure?
- How does your attitude to patients or clients change when you are under pressure?
- What challenges have you experienced that have reduced your capacity to practise in a compassionate manner?

- What have you learnt about your ability to act in a compassionate manner, which could enhance your future practice?
- How could you pass this knowledge onto colleagues or students?
- Do you feel that the culture of your practice area promotes compassionate care?
- What impact does this have on patients or clients?
- How do you feel that the nursing culture within your practice area could be enhanced further to embrace compassion in nursing?
- How could you enhance the leadership within your practice area to focus more on compassionate care?
- What resourcing issues have influenced your ability to practice in a compassionate way?
- Have you any ideas for addressing any potential issues in this area?

How do nurses work towards overcoming these challenges in practice?

CASE STUDY 8.3

Lisa – part 2

Lisa heard a friendly voice introduce herself as Jill and then the voice asked her, in a caring way, how she was.

Lisa slowly turned over, wincing at the pain as she did so, and she noticed the concern in Jill's eyes as she saw the tears run down Lisa's face. Jill had seen the involuntary wince. Lisa could see that Jill was aware of the noise and distress in the bay and this was reinforced when she said that it must be difficult to rest when there was so much going on. Jill also asked her about her pain as she was changing her intravenous bag and said that she would bring back some analgesia.

Jill returned after a few minutes and smiled again as she injected something into her cannula that she explained would help with the pain. Jill then asked her if she would find it better to move to a bay with people who were less unwell as a space had become available there. Lisa was so grateful and told Jill so. Jill put her hand on Lisa's arm and said she would arrange it. Lisa felt for the first time that someone cared about her and understood her distress and her needs. She suddenly found that she had stopped crying and was feeling a little less hopeless.

Discussion

In this second case study, Lisa was waiting for the same task-orientated approach from the next nurse. However, although the nurses were clearly very busy, Jill managed to assess Lisa's needs while she was carrying out a nursing task. Jill could see that Lisa was in pain and was distressed, and she was sensitive and empathetic enough to understand what it must feel like to be lying in that bed at that time. She came back with some analgesia and had identified a more appropriate place for Lisa to be cared for. None of this would have taken much more time than just carrying out the nursing task, but Jill's care exemplified compassion and genuine care. Jill made sure that the barriers that could have prevented her carrying out compassionate care were overcome in relation to Lisa's care. This next section discusses some potential solutions to the challenges identified in the previous section, which can prevent or reduce a compassionate approach to nursing care.

The attitude of the nurse is essential in enhancing opportunities to deliver compassionate care. Nurses need to be aware of when humour can be used in a therapeutic way and when it can be used to belittle or ridicule patients and clients. Many patients find the use of humour very therapeutic, but nurses need to be sure about when it is appropriate and when it is not. In the same way, nurses can be very stressed and distressed by the stress and distress of the people in their care and, at times, people can see this as nurses having a deep understanding of their situation. However, a stressed nurse is not really able to be therapeutic as this stress is communicated to others. This can affect team-working and patient care. Nurses need to be aware of their colleagues' stress, as well as their own, and be supportive of others who are experiencing difficult personal situations. We might need to take time off because of our personal stress or we might need to re-evaluate our reasons for wanting to nurse. Sometimes taking time out of practice to resolve our feelings and difficulties, or to come to terms with the pressures of our role, can be the only solution. Counselling and occupational health intervention can be very helpful at these times as can individual appraisals, where nurses can be encouraged to focus on their strengths and discuss areas for personal development. Clinical supervision opportunities for reflection on practice can also be helpful for individual nurses to look for ways forward.

However, sometimes there needs to be time to reflect on communication skills, cultural competence and non-judgemental attitudes outside the ward environment. Study days, ward-based action learning circles and discussion of particular challenging patient situations can all help nurses to develop different coping strategies, skills and knowledge base. Nurses should be able to identify their own learning needs and managers should ensure that there are adequate opportunities to develop the individual practice of nurses.

As can be seen in Lisa's case study (8.3), compassion can be shown in small ways at every interaction, even when nurses are busy, as this does not necessarily involve more time. Also, at quieter times, nurses should use these opportunities to go back to patients and discuss their concerns, gain their trust, and build up relationships, rather than working at the nurses' station on the ward. If working in the community, take these quieter opportunities to visit patients again, rather than going to the office to carry out administrative tasks that could, perhaps, wait.

It is essential that **the culture of the practice area** is such that compassionate care is valued and perceived as the central focus of nursing care. Effective leadership is paramount in creating this culture, because sometimes nurses do not focus on compassion in their care. They need to be empowered to practice in this way. All nurses have a leadership role, even if they are not managers, and should feel able to take a proactive lead when issues emerge in practice. We all need to challenge care that lacks compassion or which compromises professional nursing standards.

Educational and developmental opportunities that focus on compassion, dignity, cultural competence and involve people in their care could be accessed if available, or initiated if no such opportunities exist. Practice-based discussions focusing on individual patient or client needs or action learning circles around a particular learning need for nurses could also prove beneficial. In addition, empowering patients to self-care without pressurising them to do so is an under-recognised nursing skill. Discussing how to increase patient or client confidence to make decisions about their care, or their own lives, is an important learning need for many nurses. As nurses, we need to be encouraged to find ways to reintroduce patient-focused care into the more technological- and science-based tasks, so that the art of nursing remains a central tenet of practice. We all have a leadership role in creating a practice culture where care that lacks compassion is not tolerated, and where developmental opportunities exist to enhance compassionate care.

In order for any of this development to take place there needs to be strong leadership in all practice areas. Nurses need to take ownership, individually and collectively, and work as a team to ensure compassionate care is real and not merely rhetoric.

Resourcing issues: While time, resources and targets are often limiting factors in the care we give, this can sometimes be used as an excuse for inadequate care. We need to accept that time constraints and under-resourcing are often a reality in today's healthcare environment. However, we need to strive to find ways to ensure that compassionate care is built into the time available. Continuity of care is so important to patients and clients, and if this is impossible, nurses need to find ways to build relationships and rapport in the short time they have available with someone who is new in their care. There is a genuine conflict between meeting targets and delivering quality nursing care, but professional standards need to be maintained. If resourcing is inadequate for safe and compassionate care then nurses need to continue to challenge this through their organisational structure. Caring in nursing is not something we do when we have time, it should be part of what professional nursing care is considered to be. If these standards are compromised then not only do patients and clients suffer, but also it diminishes us as nurses and as a nursing profession.

While there are many potential challenges that could have a negative impact on providing compassionate care, as nurses we cannot accept this as the status quo. We have a responsibility to find innovative ways to address these challenges. Table 8.2 summarises the discussion in this section and high-lights some potential solutions for addressing these challenges.

As nurses, it is essential that we challenge practice that is not compassion-ate. Nurses need to be caring, compassionate, kind and dedicated as well as being problem-solving, analytical leaders. Sometimes it appears that the latter attributes are more highly valued than the former as the profession of nurs-ing continues to evolve. This needs to be questioned by all nurses to ensure that the compassionate core to nursing practice is not lost. As we discussed in Chapter 1, compassion and caring are inextricably linked. We have now identified the challenges to compassion and next we will focus on caring as an entity in its own right.

THOUGHTS FOR YOUR PRACTICE

- How would you identify compassionate care in your practice and the practice of others?
- How would you explain compassionate care to students?
- How can you influence the culture of your practice area to ensure that compassion is a priority?
- What strategies are used in your practice area to support nurses who are finding it difficult to cope with stressful personal experiences and the emotional demands of their role?
- If these strategies are effective, why is this?

- If these strategies could be more effective, can you think of ways in which they could be enhanced?
- What strategies are used to ensure that leadership within your practice area supports compassionate care?
- Why are these strategies effective?
- How do you ensure that you provide compassionate care during very busy times?
- How can you help others to remain compassionate even when they are busy?

KEY THEME TWO – CARING

CASE STUDY 8.4

Real life patient experience

Our baby Dexter was born full term weighing 8 lb 6 oz. He had to be put on a ventilator straight away and was immediately transferred to the neonatal unit. Over the next few days various investigations and tests were done, which gave us hope that he could make a full recovery. But then the results of his MRI scan came through; it showed that he was severely brain-damaged due to oxygen starvation. We then made the hardest decision of our lives – to ask the doctors not to resuscitate Dexter if he was unable to breathe on his own. He was just 12 days old when he died.

Throughout this distressing time the staff on the neonatal unit were outstanding. They treated Dexter with dignity throughout his short life and also after his life ended. As his parents, we were cared for with kindness and compassion. No matter how many questions we had, or how many times we asked the same thing, we were given as much time as we wanted with the consultant, paediatricians or nurses. We were always treated with courtesy and respect by everyone in the unit and they did their best to accede to our wishes (Web Site on Patient Opinion, ID 2882). Written with great courage by a father.

TABLE 8.2 Framework for compassionate practice – challenges and potential solutions

Barrier area	Challenges in relation to themes in this book	Potential solutions
Nurse attitude	• Nurse stress or anxiety • Patients mirroring the negative mood of the nurse in terms of stress or distress • Poor use of humour • Poor communication is irreversible and causes uncertainty or distress • Other behaviours that block communication • Offering false reassurance • Judgemental attitude • Belittling patient experiences or concerns • The nurse could want to distance themselves from others' distress • The nurse could have recent experiences that makes it difficult to show empathy • Moral distress of not being able to provide compassionate care • Caring overload causing desensitisation	• Nurse stress not being communicated to patients • Humour only used in a therapeutic manner • Communication skills revisited in study days and through ward-based action learning circles • Judgemental attitude and insensitive care challenged through discussion • Support of nurses who are finding it difficult to cope with personal experiences and emotional demands of their role
Culture of the organisation	• Lack of leadership that promotes dignity • Culture of the ward or practice area does not promote dignity • Privacy not maintained • Misunderstanding of patient norms and values • Different interpretation of behaviour and concerns • Person treated like an outsider • People are stereotyped • Cultural norms and values not understood	• Leadership education and support for leadership role from above and below • All nurses challenge care that lacks compassion • Practice-based discussion of ways to promote patient dignity and privacy • Education about cultural norms and cultural competence • Discuss how nursing science and tasks can be built into nursing art and patient-centred care

TABLE 8.2 (*continued*)

Barrier area	Challenges in relation to themes in this book	Potential solutions
Culture of the organisation (*cont.*)	• Emphasis on technology • Emphasis on science not art of nursing • Focus exclusively on nursing tasks • Authoritative rather than facilitative approach • Patient does not feel in control • Patient has no power and no choice • Relationships with nurses enforced • Disempowering culture of area • Patient forced to self-care or too much comfort and too little challenge • Maximises dependency • Reduces confidence to take responsibility	• Discuss how choice and control can be built into patient care • Discuss ways to encourage self-care and increase patient confidence
Resourcing issues	• Time constraints • Inadequate staffing levels • Fragmentation due to too many staff involved • Limited time to build relationships • Nurse being too busy to adapt care to actual person • Meeting targets seen as more important than dignity issues	• Accept time constraints as a real issue and discuss ways in which compassionate care can be built into the time available • Try to maintain continuity of care whenever possible • Discuss the potential conflict of meeting targets and delivering quality nursing care

Discussion

The parents in this real life patient experience clearly say that they felt 'cared for' and they relate this to the people in the neonatal unit treating them with kindness and compassion. Their baby is also treated with dignity, both when he was ill and after he died. This was such an impossibly difficult time for them, and yet they took the time to articulate what had felt so caring about their experiences in the neonatal unit. We would all hope to be treated with this degree of care when we are in such traumatic and sad situations. Unfortunately, this is sometimes not the case.

McCormack and McCance (2006) have developed a person-centred framework, which has four constructs, all of which are exemplified in this father's articulate and moving statement. They say that the **attributes of the nurse** are a prerequisite for a person-centred approach. These incorporate:

➤ professional competence;
➤ interpersonal skills, communicating on a variety of levels;
➤ clarity of beliefs and values – knowing the potential impact of these;
➤ knowing yourself (if not, how can we help others?).

The care environment or the context of care is also important in relation to:

➤ appropriate skill mix;
➤ systems that facilitate shared decision making;
➤ effective staff relationships;
➤ supportive organisational systems;
➤ sharing of power;
➤ potential for innovation and risk taking.

Person-centred processes, which involve working with patients' beliefs and values in terms of:

➤ what the patient values;
➤ how they make sense of what is happening;
➤ shared decision making;
➤ negotiation.

Finally, **outcomes**, which reflect the results of effective person-centred nursing, such as:

➤ satisfaction with care;
➤ involvement in care;
➤ feeling of well-being;
➤ shared decision making;

➤ collaborative staff relationships;
➤ transformational leadership;
➤ innovative practice that is supported.

Dexter's parents clearly felt that the nurses and the rest of the medical team had the right person-centred attributes. They were professionally competent and communicated clearly in very difficult circumstances. They were probably very experienced in dealing with this sort of traumatic situation and had clarified their own personal beliefs and how this impacted on their professional attitudes and interactions.

In addition, the care environment was a positive one and there was evidence of clear team working and effective relationships with clarity in relation to the roles they all played. The care environment and person-centred processes encouraged shared decision making and negotiation. This was based on helping the parents to make sense of what was happening and understanding what was important to them.

As a result, Dexter's parents felt involved in his care and were satisfied with the care he received. They left the unit as bereaved and highly traumatised parents, but also as people who were highly satisfied with the care they received in these dreadful circumstances.

Makin (2008) says that a nurse's role is about more than complying with legislation and policies, it is about empathy and care: 'It is not just about cure, but compassion' (p. 14). Unfortunately, Dexter could not be cured, but both he and his parents could be cared for. Makin also says that truly caring care strives to move beyond good enough care.

> Good enough is not good enough – it is mere compliance and unremarkable. We should always aim for success, which is defined by what the patients says it is. If we are satisfied with anything less than that, we are in the wrong job (Makin 2008, p. 14).

Dexter's parents obviously felt that his care had gone beyond the 'unremarkable' and was more than 'good enough' practice. For this to happen, nurses need to sometimes go beyond policies and guidelines and act with humanity to meet an individual's needs, or the needs of their loved ones.

In Scotland, there is evidence of teaching about the fundamental principles behind compassionate care. Napier University in Edinburgh, Scotland, run a Leadership in Compassionate Care initiative. Four wards are perceived as beacons of success with four senior nurses using their practice areas as learning environments for pre-registration students. Case studies and reflection are being used as learning tools to help practitioners to develop their compassionate care further (Tweddle 2007). This initiative clearly demonstrates a culture of competence where the quality of nursing leadership demonstrates a commitment within the organisation to compassionate care and to evaluating the quality of care received by patients in the four wards.

We have developed a framework for caring in nursing, which identifies what patients want from nurses and how this might be exemplified, as well as what the potential challenges might be (*see* Table 8.3).

This framework for caring is based on areas that are perceived as important within the Confidence in Caring document (DOH 2008), as discussed in Chapter 1, which include care provider, care partner, champion and coordinator (*see* Table 8.3, column 1). In addition, the framework includes other aspects that we believe are important to patients, such as getting to know the patient or client, wanting to ease their distress and enabling or empowering them to become partners in their care. We have identified in column 2 how this caring might be obvious to patients or clients, but we have also identified some potential challenges to nurses in demonstrating this care in practice (*see* column 3).

The next section discusses how nurses can ensure that caring remains central to their practice and how they can continue to challenge a lack of caring in their own practice and that of others.

How do we ensure that caring is central within our nursing practice?

CASE STUDY 8.5

Jackie had been involved in Emily's care at her home for the past few months and the deterioration in her health and ability to take an active part in her care had happened quite fast. Jackie felt very sad for Emily. They were of a similar age and multiple sclerosis had taken so much away from Emily. Jackie could not imagine how she would have coped with Emily's life and what it had become.

Jackie had a close professional relationship with Emily that was therapeutic and supportive, and they had talked many times about quality of life and when life could become unbearable. Jackie was aware that their views around end-of-life care were different and this had not impacted on their relationship. Jackie had strong religious views and believed that life was sacrosanct and that a person had no right to interfere with the way that life had been planned for you. Emily, on the other hand, felt that if her quality of life became too compromised and her distress became too great for her, then she would want someone to help her in her distress, even if this meant that her life was shorter because of any medication that was prescribed.

On this particular day Jackie realised that Emily had come to the point that what she feared most was happening. She was finding it harder to breathe and she was very frightened. Jackie held her hand and tried to give her strength through talking calmly and quietly. She phoned the doctor who came quickly because they knew that Emily's condition was deteriorating fast. The doctor, Andrea, spoke to Jackie outside the room, once she had seen and spoken to Emily. Andrea said that she felt that Emily needed to be prescribed some sedation to try to alleviate her distress and increase her drowsiness so that she would be less aware of her increasing symptoms. Jackie was convinced that this would also have the effect of shortening Emily's life, and as she did not believe that Emily was actually in physical pain, she did not feel that this was justifiable. Andrea had talked about distressing symptoms and the need to alleviate these. Jackie did not feel that she wanted to be put in the position of administering this sedation because she felt this would contravene her religious beliefs, but she was aware that she was the only person on duty over this weekend that would be able to do so.

Discussion

Obviously, Jackie had a very close relationship with Emily and felt great empathy for her situation. Her care up until this point had been exemplary and therapeutic. However, there had been increasing evidence of the fact that they had different moral beliefs. As Emily's condition deteriorated, these differences in beliefs became more pronounced. This eventually caused an impasse at the most vulnerable stage of Emily's life. Jackie should have been acting as her champion and advocate, but was unable to do so because of her own beliefs.

Jackie had insufficient knowledge of end-of-life care and that pain manifests itself in many ways, which included the distress that Emily was clearly feeling. If she had been more up to date with current medication strategies for people at the end of their lives, then she should have re-evaluated her own beliefs and seen Emily's needs as paramount. In doing so, she would have been practising more in line with the philosophies that underpin professional codes of practice in relation to patient-centred care. She was not

TABLE 8.3 Framework for caring in nursing – evidence and challenges

Column 1 What patients want	Column 2 Evidence of caring	Column 3 Challenges to caring
Care provider (DOH 2008)	• Professional appearance and behaviour • Competent • Knowledgeable • Compassionate • Provides holistic, timely, seamless care and information	• Nurses appearing professional • Keeping up to date – knowledge and competence • Not working within codes of professional practice • Lack of professional support and supervision • Credibility of information available • Seeing the patient as a whole person with individual needs
Care partner (DOH 2008)	• Works with patients and relatives to plan care • Gives constant feedback and reports • Helps them to navigate the health and social care system	• Not seeking or responding to patient or user feedback • Time needed to work in partnership with patients or clients – planning and feedback • Constant change within health and social care systems
Champion (DOH 2008)	• Puts their interests first • Protects them when they are vulnerable	• Conflict of interests • Inappropriate prioritisation • Not realising when people are vulnerable • Not appreciating the importance of their role as an advocate
Coordinator (DOH 2008)	• Constant • Accessible • Accountable for communicating the plan • Monitors the delivery of care	• Too many people involved • Little continuity of care • Too many roles leading to fragmentation • Lack of effective evaluation of care
Getting to know them and being with them	• Showing interest in them • Liking them • Valuing them • Respecting them as people • Spending time with them	• Some patients or clients may challenge our personal beliefs/values • Nurses might actively avoid spending time with some people

TABLE 8.3 (*continued*)

Column 1	Column 2	Column 3
What patients want	Evidence of caring	Challenges to caring
Wanting to ease distress	• Doing things for them • Committed to high quality care • Showing concern for them • Being compassionate	• Difficult balance between comfort and challenge • Sometimes quicker to do things for people than spending time helping them to become independent • Challenge of being caring and providing high quality care within reduced resources
Enabling	• Increasing self-esteem and self-belief • Empowering them to be more in control	• Different age-related beliefs about empowerment • Different cultures view empowerment in different ways • Encouraging 'self-care' as a cheaper option

viewing Emily's needs holistically, nor was she listening to what was important for Emily.

Jackie had a clear conflict of interest because she wanted to provide sensitive care for Emily, but her own beliefs took precedence when Emily was at her most vulnerable. Some patients and clients do challenge our norms and values and we need to have sufficient self-awareness to be able to predict potential areas of conflict. Where these conflicts are insurmountable for a particular nurse, strategies must be developed in advance as a team. Nurses need to be advocates for their patients and clients, but also support and empower individuals in making decisions about their care.

The individual attitude of the nurse is paramount, as discussed in the paragraph above. However, the culture of the practice area is important in providing care that is genuinely caring. For example, other nurses working in the locality could have worked collaboratively to meet Emily's needs if Jackie's beliefs made this impossible for her. Other nurses might have needed to have become involved in Emily's care before this crucial stage, to provide continuity of care and reduce fragmentation to ensure that her needs were met. However, this would need to have been achieved within the resources available.

THOUGHTS FOR YOUR PRACTICE

- What attributes do you feel you possess that demonstrate to patients, clients, colleagues and students that you are professionally competent in the way you care?
- In what way does your practice area encourage the facilitation of patient-centred care?
- Think of an example from practice where you worked closely with a patient or client and based your care on their beliefs and values.
- Evaluate this experience and think about ways in which you could share this learning with colleagues and students.
- How do you know that patients perceive your practice as caring?
- Can you think of ways in which your personal beliefs could come into conflict with meeting patients' or clients' needs?
- How would you address this in practice?

How can we continue to challenge a lack of caring in our own practice and that of others?

CASE STUDY 8.6

Real life patient experience

We recently came to Macclesfield Hospital as an emergency; the staff, care and treatment in A&E were brilliant. After transfer to ward 8, I can only say that they treated both my father and myself with the utmost care and compassion during our stay. The staff looked after my father so well, I couldn't have asked for more. They were the same with all the patients, and paid particular attention to people's privacy and dignity.

They also looked after me as the carer; nothing was too much trouble. (Web Site on Patient Opinion, ID 3149)

Discussion

The daughter in this real life patient experience clearly felt cared for as a relative and carer, as well as feeling that her father had been well cared for. She mentions, specifically, that nurses were compassionate and treated her father with dignity and respected his need for privacy. The fact that they interacted with her in a caring way was also obviously very important to her. Therefore, individual nurses were caring, and there was a culture of caring within the ward, which meant that time constraints and resourcing did not negatively impact on this care.

These areas of potential challenge to caring practice were not obvious to the author of this comment, despite the fact that the nurses were undoubtedly very busy, which could have resulted in a less caring culture. As nurses, we feel that we need to continue to challenge a potential lack of caring in others and ourselves.

Firstly, in relation to **nurses' attitudes, as individuals**, we need to ensure that we take personal responsibility for our learning and identify the gaps in our knowledge, or where our knowledge is not up to date. This means requesting or attending study days and actively seeking other opportunities for learning. We need to make sure that we understand our codes of professional practice and what they mean for our own areas of practice. These can be useful tools for us in providing quality care, as managers tend to be risk-averse and do not want complaints or negative publicity from poor patient or client feedback, or from cases where nurses' practice is called into question. Decisions about nursing care need to be made using clear evidence, a team approach, holistic assessment and critical review, as these exemplify the background to caring practice. As individuals, we need to possess a high level of self-awareness that enables us to question our own practice and beliefs and allows us to have team discussions on difficult ethical situations. Every effort needs to be made to focus clearly on the patient or client, and team discussions and peer supervision can help us to carry on challenging ways in which care could be compromised. Some patients and clients can be harder for us to like, or identify with, and we need to focus on what we have in common, rather than what makes us different. Our colleagues might provide useful insights for us to develop our practice in this way. We also need to be aware of the fact that, although we want to appear caring, we could be over-nurturing and people could then become over-dependent on us. This could have a negative effect on their self-belief and just how effective they can be themselves.

Secondly, in terms of the **culture of the organisation**, it is important to understand that people want nurses to act and dress in a professional manner, as this engenders feelings of trust in us and feeling safe in our care. This often requires a team approach to identify clear standards of practice for our practice area. Clinical supervision should be available on a regular basis as a tool for reflection and development. Feedback from clients, patients and their carers should stimulate us to challenge areas of our practice that are less caring. We need to work in partnership with people in our care to identify ways to continuously improve our care, and this needs to be within a constantly changing healthcare environment. We need to regularly challenge norms and values and our level of cultural competence to ensure that this remains the case.

Thirdly, in terms of **resourcing**, we need to challenge inadequate resources that have a negative impact on our caring capacity. This involves understanding that while we could always benefit from greater resources, the continuity of care, clarity about 'who does what for whom' and a focus on quality driven initiatives will always be important for nursing care, to ensure the spotlight remains firmly focused on both quality and care.

Having identified the challenges for caring within the framework in Table 8.3, we have taken these challenges further by presenting some potential solutions in the discussion above. These we have drawn together in Table 8.4, which we hope offers you an overview of these important issues.

TABLE 8.4 Framework for caring in nursing – challenges and potential solutions

Challenge area	Challenges to caring	Potential solutions
Nurse attitude	• Keeping up to date – knowledge and competence • Not working within codes of professional practice • Credibility of information available • Seeing the patient as a whole person with individual needs • Conflict of interests • Inappropriate prioritisation and decision making • Not realising when people are vulnerable • Not appreciating the importance of our role as an advocate • Some patients or clients may challenge our personal beliefs/values • Nurses might actively avoid spending time with some people • Difficult balance between comfort and challenge • Sometimes quicker to do things for people than spending time helping them to become independent	• Personal responsibility for learning and identifying areas of development • Access to study days and practice-based discussion opportunities • Familiarity with codes of practice and content • Decisions made on knowledge, understanding and competence in holistic assessment • Self-awareness • Team discussion of ethical dilemmas in practice • Effective critical review skills • Nurse is aware of need for evidence-based practice • Prioritisation of patients' needs • Not losing sight of the person as a vulnerable individual, case scenarios and supervision to challenge practice and norms and values • Revisit personal values and beliefs • Prioritising building of relationships and time spent with patients whenever possible, particularly with people who we find hard to like • Act as advocate and provide emotional comfort where necessary, but understand the importance of challenge and empowerment when appropriate

(continued)

TABLE 8.4 (*continued*)

Challenge area	Challenges to caring	Potential solutions
Culture of the organisation	• Nurses appearing professional • Lack of professional support and supervision • Not seeking or responding to patient or user feedback • Time needed to work in partnership with patients or clients – planning and feedback • Constant change within health and social care systems • Lack of effective evaluation of care • Different age-related beliefs about empowerment • Different cultures view empowerment in different ways	• Standards of dress and performance clearly understood • Access to clinical supervision and individual support on an ongoing basis • Actively seek user feedback via a range of strategies • Act on feedback received as appropriate • Focus on working in partnership with patients and encourage others to do the same • Work as a team to ensure that time is used effectively • Constantly re-evaluate need for change and be proactive about anticipating change • Encourage ourselves, students and colleagues to challenge accepted norms and values • Encourage cultural competence within every practice area through focused discussion
Resourcing issues	• Too many people involved • Little continuity of care • Too many roles leading to fragmentation • Challenge of being caring and providing high quality care within reduced resources • Encouraging 'self-care' as a cheaper option	• Actively seek ways to reduce the number of carers involved and to promote continuity of care • Clarity about the different roles in practice and what they bring to care • Focus on quality care despite reduced resources • Ensure that self-care is needs based and do not use self-care as a way to reduce care needs

THOUGHTS FOR YOUR PRACTICE

- How do you ensure that you keep yourself professionally up to date?
- How do you try to identify gaps in your knowledge and skills that you did not know were there?
- What opportunities are there in your practice area to regularly review how you and your colleagues work as a team?
- What strategies are used in your practice area for you and your colleagues to share, challenge and learn from each other's experiences?
- What methods do you use to actively seek patient or client feedback?
- Do you feel that you act positively to address issues raised in feedback?
- Could you further enhance response to feedback to develop practice in your area?
- How do you ensure that you remain genuinely caring within limited resources?

SUMMARY – LINKS TO COMPASSION AND CARING

We hope that this book has opened new challenges for your nursing practice in relation to how your care can remain compassionate and genuinely caring in the resource-driven environments in which we all practise nowadays. We have identified particular themes that we think are fundamental to compassionate and caring nursing practice. We have tried to address the challenges that exist in relation to caring for patients and clients in the manner that we would want our loved ones to be cared for, and how we would want to be cared for ourselves.

We need to continue to challenge ourselves, and support and challenge our colleagues, to practise with compassion. We need to act as role models and specifically discuss compassion with our students and new members of staff. This will ensure that the culture of our practice area upholds compassionate care as a central component of the nursing environment we are part of. We also need to act as gatekeepers of our profession to ensure that this is the case.

As nurses, we must believe in compassionate caring and remember, as von Dietze and Orb (2000) say: 'compassionate care is not simplistically about taking away another person's pain or suffering, but is about entering into that person's experience so as to share their burden in solidarity with them and hence enabling them to retain their independence and dignity' (p. 169). They go on to say that this 'is more than a principle or ingredient of care . . . but is part of the core of that which defines successful professional care' (p. 173).

We were profoundly affected by the following poem, as it epitomises, for us, the very reason why we feel so passionately about compassion and caring. The poem is simply called 'Kate'. The author was in hospital and unable to speak, but was occasionally seen to write. After her death, her hospital locker was emptied and this poem was found (Carver and Liddiard 1978, pp. ix–xi).

Kate

What do you see nurses, what do you see?
Are you thinking when you are looking at me?
A crabbit old woman not very wise
Uncertain of habit with far-away eyes
Who dribbles her food and makes no reply
When you say in a loud voice 'I do wish you'd try'
Who seems not to notice the things that you do
And forever is losing a stocking or shoe
Who, unresisting or not, lets you do as you will
With bathing or feeding the long day to fill
Is that what you're thinking, is that what you see?
Then open your eyes nurse, you're not looking at me.
I'll tell you who I am as I sit here so still!
As I rise at your bidding, as I eat at your will.
I'm a small child of 10 with a father and mother
Brothers and sisters, who loved one another.
A young girl of 16 with wings on her feet
Dreaming that soon now a lover she'll meet
A bride soon at 20 – my heart gives a leap
Remembering the vows that I promised to keep.
At 25 now I have young of my own
Who need me to build a secure happy home.
A woman of 30, my young now grow fast
Bound to each other with ties that should last.
At 40, my young sons have grown and are gone
But my man's beside me to see I don't mourn.
At 50 once more babies play around my knee
Again we know children, my loved one and me.

Dark days are upon me, my husband is dead

I look at the future, I shudder with dread

For my young are all rearing young of their own.

And I think of the years and the love that I've known;

I'm an old woman now and nature is cruel

'Tis her jest to make old age look like a fool

The body it crumbles, grace and vigour depart

There now is a stone where once I had a heart.

But inside this old carcass a young girl still dwells

And now and again my battered heart swells

I remember the joys, I remember the pain

And I'm loving and living life over again

I think of the years all too few – gone too fast

And accept the stark fact that nothing can last.

So open your eyes nurses, open and see

Not a crabbit old woman; look closer – see ME.'

All Kate wanted was for the nurses involved in her care to see her as an individual person and show her more respect, dignity, empathy, sensitivity and all the other central tenets that comprise compassionate and caring nursing practice.

REFERENCES

Carver V, Liddiard P. *An Ageing Population*. Kent: Hodder and Stoughton in association with Open University Press; 1978.

Department of Health. *Confidence in Caring: a framework for best practice*. London: Department of Health; 2008.

Goleman D. *Destructive Emotions and How We Can Overcome Them*. London: Bloomsbury; 2004.

Hem M, Heggen K. Is compassion central to nursing practice? *Contemp Nurse*. 2004; **17**: 19–31.

McCabe C. Nurse-patient communication: an exploration of patients' experiences. *J Clin Nurs*. 2004; **13**(1): 41–9.

McCormack B, McCance T. The development of a framework for person-centred nursing. *J Adv Nurs*. 2006; **56**(5): 472–9.

Makin A. There is a lot more to nursing than just complying to legislation and policies. *Nurs Times*. 2008; **104**(6): 14.

Tweddle L. Compassion on the curriculum. *Nurs Times*. 2007; **103**(38): 18–19.

von Dietze E, Orb A. Compassionate care: a moral dimension of nursing. *Nursing Inquiry*. 2000; **7**(3): 166–74.

Williams A, Irurita V. Therapeutic and non-therapeutic interpersonal interactions: the patient's perspective. *J Clin Nurs*. 2004; **13**(7): 806–15.

www.patientopinion.org.uk/opinion.aspx?opinionID=2882
www.patientopinion.org.uk/opinion.aspx?opinionID=3149
www.patientopinion.org.uk/opinion.aspx?opinionID=7846

Index

Text in tables is denoted by entries in **bold**.